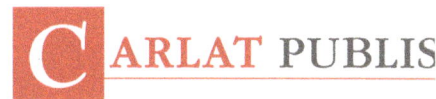 

Child Medication Fact Book
for Psychiatric Practice

Joshua Feder, MD
Associate Clinical Professor at University of California at San Diego School of Medicine

Elizabeth Tien, MD
Supervising Psychiatrist at the Mental Health Service Corps

Talia Puzantian, PharmD, BCPP
Associate Professor at Keck Graduate Institute School of Pharmacy, Claremont, CA

Published by Carlat Publishing, LLC
PO Box 626, Newburyport, MA 01950

Copyright © 2018 All Rights Reserved.

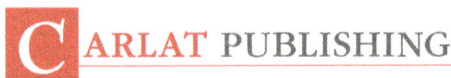

Child Medication Fact Book
For Psychiatric Practice

Published by Carlat Publishing, LLC
PO Box 626, Newburyport, MA 01950

Publisher and Editor-in-Chief: Daniel J. Carlat, MD
Deputy Editor: Talia Puzantian, PharmD, BCPP
Executive Editor: Janice Jutras

All rights reserved. This book is protected by copyright.

This CME/CE activity is intended for psychiatrists, psychiatric nurses, psychologists, and other health care professionals with an interest in mental health. The Carlat CME Institute is accredited by the Accreditation Council for Continuing Medical Education to provide continuing medical education for physicians. Carlat CME Institute is approved by the American Psychological Association to sponsor continuing education for psychologists. Carlat CME Institute maintains responsibility for this program and its content. Carlat CME Institute designates this enduring material educational activity for a maximum of eight (8) AMA PRA Category 1 Credits™ or 8 CE for psychologists. Physicians or psychologists should claim credit commensurate only with the extent of their participation in the activity. The American Board of Psychiatry and Neurology has reviewed the *Child Medication Fact Book for Psychiatric Practice* and has approved this program as part of a comprehensive Self-Assessment and CME Program, which is mandated by ABMS as a necessary component of maintenance of certification. CME quizzes must be taken online at www.thecarlatreport.com or http://thecarlatcmeinstitute.com/self-assessment (for ABPN SA course subscribers).

To order, visit www.thecarlatreport.com
or call (866) 348-9279

1 2 3 4 5 6 7 8 9 10

ISBN #: 978-0-9975106-8-3

PRINTED IN THE UNITED STATES OF AMERICA

Table of Contents

Introduction 5

General Tips on Child and Adolescent Psychopharmacology 7
Note: Some medications, eg guanfacine, are covered in more than one chapter; however, the fact sheets are listed only in one of those chapters.

ADHD Medications 11
Amphetamine (Adzenys XR-ODT, Dyanavel XR, Evekeo) Fact Sheet 16
Atomoxetine (Strattera) Fact Sheet [G] 17
Clonidine (Catapres, Kapvay) Fact Sheet [G] 18
Dexmethylphenidate (Focalin) Fact Sheet [G] 19
Dextroamphetamine (Dexedrine) Fact Sheet [G] 20
Guanfacine (Intuniv, Tenex) Fact Sheet [G] 21
Lisdexamfetamine (Vyvanse) Fact Sheet 22
Methamphetamine (Desoxyn) Fact Sheet [G] 23
Methylphenidate IR (Ritalin) Fact Sheet [G] 24
Methylphenidate ER (Concerta, Ritalin-SR and LA) Fact Sheet [G] 25
Methylphenidate Transdermal (Daytrana) Fact Sheet 26
Mixed Amphetamine Salts (Adderall) Fact Sheet [G] 27

Antidepressants 29
Bupropion (Wellbutrin) Fact Sheet [G] 32
Citalopram (Celexa) Fact Sheet [G] 33
Desvenlafaxine (Pristiq) Fact Sheet [G] 34
Duloxetine (Cymbalta) Fact Sheet [G] 35
Escitalopram (Lexapro) Fact Sheet [G] 36
Fluoxetine (Prozac) Fact Sheet [G] 37
Fluvoxamine (Luvox) Fact Sheet [G] 38
Mirtazapine (Remeron) Fact Sheet [G] 39
Paroxetine (Paxil, Pexeva) Fact Sheet [G] 40
Selegiline Transdermal (EMSAM) Fact Sheet 41
Sertraline (Zoloft) Fact Sheet [G] 42
Trazodone Fact Sheet [G] 43
Tricyclic Antidepressants (TCAs) Fact Sheet [G] 44
Venlafaxine (Effexor XR) Fact Sheet [G] 45

Antipsychotics 47
Aripiprazole (Abilify) Fact Sheet [G] 51
Asenapine (Saphris) Fact Sheet 52
Chlorpromazine (Thorazine) Fact Sheet [G] 53
Clozapine (Clozaril) Fact Sheet [G] 54
Haloperidol (Haldol) Fact Sheet [G] 55
Lurasidone (Latuda) Fact Sheet 56

Olanzapine (Zyprexa) Fact Sheet [G] 57
Paliperidone (Invega) Fact Sheet [G] 58
Perphenazine (Trilafon) Fact Sheet [G] 59
Quetiapine (Seroquel) Fact Sheet [G] 60
Risperidone (Risperdal) Fact Sheet [G] 61
Ziprasidone (Geodon) Fact Sheet [G] 62
Long-Acting Injectable (LAI) Antipsychotics 63

Anxiolytics and Hypnotics 67
Antihistamines (Diphenhydramine, Doxylamine, Hydroxyzine) Fact Sheet [G] 72
Buspirone (BuSpar) Fact Sheet [G] 73
Clonazepam (Klonopin) Fact Sheet [G] 74
Lorazepam (Ativan) Fact Sheet [G] 75
Prazosin (Minipress) Fact Sheet [G] 76
Propranolol (Inderal) Fact Sheet [G] 77

Complementary Treatments 79
L-Methylfolate (Deplin) Fact Sheet 82
Magnesium Fact Sheet 83
Melatonin Fact Sheet 84
N-Acetylcysteine (NAC) Fact Sheet 85
Omega-3 Fatty Acids (Fish Oil) Fact Sheet.. 86
S-Adenosyl-L-Methionine (SAMe) Fact Sheet.. 87
St. John's Wort Fact Sheet 88
Vitamin D Fact Sheet 89

Mood Stabilizers.. 91
Carbamazepine (Tegretol) Fact Sheet [G] 93
Lamotrigine (Lamictal) Fact Sheet [G] 94
Lithium (Lithobid) Fact Sheet [G] 95
Oxcarbazepine (Trileptal) Fact Sheet [G] 96
Valproic Acid (Depakote) Fact Sheet [G] 97

Substance Use Medications 99
Acamprosate (Campral) Fact Sheet [G]...102
Buprenorphine (Buprenex, Probuphine, Sublocade) Fact Sheet [G]...........103
Buprenorphine/Naloxone (Suboxone) Fact Sheet [G] 104
Disulfiram (Antabuse) Fact Sheet [G] 105
Methadone (Methadose) Fact Sheet [G] 106
Naloxone (Evzio, Narcan Nasal Spray) Fact Sheet [G] 107
Naltrexone (ReVia, Vivitrol) Fact Sheet [G] 108
Nicotine Gum/Lozenge (Nicorette) Fact Sheet [G] 109
Nicotine Inhaled (Nicotrol Inhaler) Fact Sheet...110
Nicotine Nasal Spray (Nicotrol NS) Fact Sheet 111
Nicotine Patch (Nicoderm CQ) Fact Sheet [G] 112
Varenicline (Chantix) Fact Sheet..113

Appendices ... 115
Appendix A: Blood Pressure Parameters for Children ... 115
Appendix B: Growth and Body Mass Index Charts ... 119
Appendix C: Abnormal Involuntary Movement Scale (AIMS) ... 123
Appendix D: Guidelines for Informed Consent ... 126
Appendix E: Drug Interactions in Psychiatry ... 127
Appendix F: Schedules of Controlled Substances ... 134
Appendix G: Lab Monitoring for Psychiatric Medications ... 135
Appendix H: Pharmacogenetic Testing Recommendations ... 136
Appendix I: Medications in Pregnancy and Lactation Risk Information ... 138

List of Tables
Table 1: ADHD Medications ... 13
Table 2: Antidepressants ... 30
Table 3: First-Generation Antipsychotics ... 49
Table 4: Second-Generation Antipsychotics ... 49
Table 5: Long-Acting Injectable Antipsychotics ... 64
Table 6: Anxiolytics and Hypnotics ... 69
Table 6.1: Benzodiazepine Dosage Equivalencies ... 71
Table 7: Complementary Treatments ... 81
Table 8: Mood Stabilizers ... 92
Table 9: Substance Use and Dependence Medications ... 100

Index ... 143

Introduction

HOW TO USE THIS BOOK

Medication information is presented in three ways in this book.

Chapter introductions: These are guides to general therapeutic categories of child psychopharmacology. There is natural overlap between these areas; however, we hope that our groupings are convenient for quick reference in everyday office practice.

Medication fact sheets: In-depth prescribing information for select medications (not all psychiatric medications are covered). There are 70 medication fact sheets in this book. Medications that fall into more than one category are included in each applicable chapter table, but each medication has only one fact sheet (placed in the chapter where we believe the medication is most commonly used). We have included most of the commonly prescribed and newer medications for which there are data and experience in children. These fact sheets include dosing, indications and common uses (both on and off label), side effects, mechanisms of action, recommendations for clinical monitoring, evidence, clinical pearls, and fun facts.

Quick-scan medication tables: These are located after the chapter introduction for each therapeutic category and list the very basics: generic and brand names, FDA-approved indications, strengths available, starting doses, and target doses. These tables contain most of the commonly prescribed psychiatric medications in pediatric practice.

CATEGORIES OF MEDICATIONS

We did our best to categorize medications rationally. However, in some cases a medication can fall into more than one category. In such cases, we placed the medication's fact sheet in the therapeutic category for which it is most often used. If you're having trouble finding a medication in a particular section, look in the index to find its page number.

MORE ON THE MEDICATION FACT SHEETS

The goal of these fact sheets is to provide need-to-know information that can be easily and quickly absorbed during a busy day of seeing patients. An important goal, therefore, is that all the information should fit on a single page. Please refer to the *PDR (Physicians' Desk Reference)* when you need more in-depth information.

- For the most part, each fact sheet contains the following information:
- Both the brand and generic names.
- Generic availability, denoted with a [G] or (G).
- FDA-approved indications in kids and in adults.
- Off-label uses. We list the more common off-label uses, based on both the medical literature and our own clinical experience. Just because we list a potential use does not imply that we endorse a medication as being particularly effective for that use. We are simply alerting you to the fact that there is some evidence for efficacy or at least reports of use.
- Dosage forms, along with available strengths.
- Dosage guidance. We provide recommendations on how to dose medications; these are derived from a variety of sources, including package inserts, clinical trials, and common clinical practice. In other words, don't be surprised when our dosing instructions are at odds with what you find in the *PDR* or other sources such as RxList.
- Lab monitoring recommendations. We include the usual routine monitoring measures for each medication. Of course, you may need to think beyond the "routine" if the clinical picture warrants it.
- Cost information. Pricing information for a 1-month supply of a common dosing regimen was obtained from the website GoodRx (*www.goodrx.com*), accessed in May 2018. These are the prices patients would have to pay if they had no insurance. Because of wide variations in price depending on the pharmacy, in this edition of the *Child Medication Fact Book* we list price categories rather than the price in dollars. The categories are:
  - $: Inexpensive: <$50/month
  - $$: Moderate: $50–$100/month
  - $$$: Expensive: $100–$200/month
  - $$$$: Very expensive: $200–$500/month
  - $$$$$: Extremely expensive: >$500/month

  Many patients have some type of insurance and are therefore not going to pay retail price, but rather a co-pay, which is usually less expensive. However, off-label uses of medications in child psychiatry are often not covered by insurance. Also, even when covered, the co-pays for medication can be high, particularly for high-deductible insurance plans. With no clear source for accurately predicting a co-pay, you can use the retail price as a clue. Meds that are very inexpensive may

require no co-pay, while the most expensive drugs will either require a very expensive co-pay, or, more likely, will not be covered at all without an onerous pre-authorization process.
- Side effects information. We break down side effects into "most common" vs "rare but serious" side effects. We generally define "most common" side effects as those occurring in at least 5% of patients in clinical trials, and which were at least double the rate of the placebo group. Such information is usually found in tables in the drugs' package inserts. We also used post-marketing clinical experience as a guide in determining which side effects were common enough to make the list.
- Mechanism of action. While the mechanism of action is not well-established for most psychiatric drugs, we thought it would be important to report the mechanisms most commonly cited.
- Pharmacokinetics, with a focus on drug metabolism and/or half-life.
- Drug interactions.
- Evidence and clinical pearls, which typically comment on the evidence base for use in children and the advantages or disadvantages of a medication in comparison to others in its therapeutic category, tips for dosing or avoiding side effects, types of patients who seem to benefit the most, reports about off-label use, and so forth.
- Fun facts.
- Lastly, our bottom-line summary or assessment for that particular medication.

APPENDICES

Please note that in these appendices we include a number of medications that are not generally used in children but are listed for completeness.
- Blood pressure parameters for children. A guide for clinicians, in particular for children on stimulant medication.
- Growth and body mass index charts. These are also helpful in our work as we track the growth and development of our patients.
- Abnormal Involuntary Movement Scale (AIMS). While we wish to avoid unneeded use of antipsychotic medications and others that might cause tardive dyskinesia, the AIMS helps us to monitor for such side effects.
- Informed consent guidelines. This topic can be particularly complicated in child and adolescent psychiatry, so here we offer guidelines for clinicians to navigate this process.
- Drug interactions in psychiatry. While we do provide some information on drug interactions in the fact sheets, this appendix features a more extensive discussion of the topic, as well as a table of interactions for commonly prescribed drugs.
- Schedules of controlled substances. Just in case you can't remember which drugs are in which DEA schedule or what each schedule means, we have you covered with a handy table.
- Lab monitoring for psychiatric medications. We've included a short quick-reference table listing the medications that require laboratory monitoring, along with the labs you should consider ordering.
- Pharmacogenetic testing recommendations. Although we do not feel that pharmacogenetic testing has reached a stage of routine clinical utility, we've added a brief section providing some basic information.
- Pregnancy and lactation risk information. The risks and benefits of using psychiatric medications in pregnancy and breastfeeding are not as simple or clear as the previously used "ABCDX" categories might suggest. The new Pregnancy and Lactation Labeling Rule (PLLR) has been implemented by the FDA, resulting in a more detailed narrative describing available risk data instead of the letter category designation. Rather than putting this information in the fact sheets, we have a separate section in the appendices devoted to the topic.

FINANCIAL DISCLOSURES

Drs. Feder, Tien, and Puzantian have disclosed that they have no relevant relationships or financial interests in any commercial company pertaining to the information provided in this book.

DISCLAIMER

The medication information in this book was formulated with a reasonable standard of care and in conformity with professional standards in the field of child and adolescent psychiatry. Medication prescribing decisions are complex, and you should use these fact sheets as only one of many possible sources of medication information. This information is not a substitute for informed medical care. This book is intended for use by licensed professionals only.

If you have any comments or corrections, please let us know by writing to us at info@thecarlatreport.com or Carlat Publishing, P. O. Box 626, Newburyport, MA 01950.

General Tips on Child and Adolescent Psychopharmacology

Over the course of a career, most of us realize that pediatric psychopharmacology is more art than science, and that much of the knowledge we've acquired over the years has come from our work with patients after completing residency and fellowship. Here are some hard-won tips and pearls that you might find useful in your practice.

ASSESSMENT, DIAGNOSIS, AND CASE CONCEPTUALIZATION

- **Target symptoms are king.** Most patients come to us with mixed symptoms from several diagnostic categories. Depression, for example, takes on myriad shapes in different patients, with the result that this one diagnosis can seem like many. While formal diagnosis is helpful for insurance and school advocacy, for treatment it is usually more practical to list and prioritize target symptoms. During the workup and ongoing follow-up, it is very helpful to have a running list of all the presenting and ongoing target symptoms, circling the ones that are the current focus. For instance, in one patient you might be targeting substance use, mood instability, and impulsivity, circling all three, while leaving issues of poor grades, tics, and peer relationships on the list but uncircled—intending to focus on them a bit down the line. Another patient with the same set of symptoms might have different issues to target.
- **Meds are the tail, not the dog.** Medications can be very helpful at times, even life-saving, but they cannot make up for an inadequate overall plan or placement. If a child is laboring under challenging or outright abusive situations at home or school, pills do not fix that. For instance, a teen with moderate autism spectrum disorder was brought in for a medication evaluation for irritability and "acting out." On evaluation, his treatment plan included "training for pre-vocational skills"—and his acting out turned out to be in part a rebellion from years of being subjugated to tasks such as sorting silverware. The answer in this case was to rethink the goals that had been imposed on the patient as part of the treatment plan, and not to provide chemical restraint.
- **Informed consent is your friend.** Use informed consent—diagnosis, target symptoms, discussion of options, etc—to guide rational treatment. See the appendices for additional tips on this process.
- **Good care demands time.** You know this, and you are probably fighting for time—time to see the patient; talk to family, therapists, and teachers; review records; call labs; and whatever else you need to do to care for your patient. When we are taken to task about care, we are asked such things as: "Did you contact the school?" "Did you call the lab?" We need time to do these things, and we deserve to be paid for that time too. Advocate for more time for all the elements of patient care.
- **Keep development in mind.** One of the joys of our field is that we have the opportunity to see the range of changes that occur developmentally and to explain to parents, teachers, and colleagues that these are not "symptoms." For example, an active toddler does not necessarily have ADHD. A school-aged child with a vivid fantasy life is usually not psychotic.
- **Always consider the possibility of abuse.** It is estimated that 1/4 to 1/3 of girls and 1/6 of boys are sexually abused before age 18; always assess for sexual and physical abuse as well as neglect. Ask about discipline and about supervision as a part of your formal assessment. Parents often want help in managing their frustration (and perhaps their own difficulties with mood, substances, etc), and this is an opportunity to be of great help.
- **Drug and substance use are common.** We should always ask teens (and even tweens) about substance use. This includes the usual things like tobacco, alcohol, marijuana, and other drugs; prescribed medications such as stimulants and opiates; and now also non-prescribed opiates, CBD, and newer drugs of abuse. In addition, consider household substances not yet or newly criminalized such as Spice and others.
- **We may save more lives with a safety check than anything else we do.** Talk with parents about locking up alcohol, medications (including OTCs), and hazardous household products. We often add an admonition to lock up guns, ropes, cords, and sharp knives as part of a safety check. Ask about sunscreen, hydration, seat belts, and driving habits of the patient and the family.

MEDICATION MANAGEMENT AND MONITORING TARGET SYMPTOMS

- **One change at a time.** Try to make only one medication change at a time. Starting two medications at once, for example, can make it hard to tell which one is easing symptoms and which one is causing side effects. There will be exceptions, particularly in more urgent situations; however, it is best to try to be parsimonious and patient.
- **Start low and go slow.** While making small changes may take patience and reassurance, rapid or large changes in medications often lead to untoward side effects and aborted medication trials. It is helpful to tell families, especially if they are hesitant about medication, that we want to use the lowest dose that is effective; therefore, the best first result is to see no change in symptoms and no side effects, because we've used so little medication. From here, we bring up the dose gradually so we can see the results.
- **Take it down (slowly) if it doesn't work.** There is little point in keeping a medication at a robust dose if it is not having a clear positive impact. We often see people who have stayed on medications more out of habit than anything else. Get

rid of unneeded medications, but do it gradually. The medication may in fact be helping, or perhaps a combination is important (eg, in classic bipolar disorder).

- **Beware regression to the mean.** We often see people when things are difficult; however, many symptoms will wax and wane as part of their natural course. If we start a medication when a particular symptom is at its worst, we may ascribe the subsequent improvement to our intervention, when the symptom would have gotten better anyway. The reverse is also true: When a symptom worsens, we may automatically attribute it to a life event or to a medication change.
- **Placebo effects are common.** Hope and faith are good things and might result in positive results from an otherwise ineffective medication. If a positive response diminishes after about 6 weeks, it may have been mostly a placebo effect.
- **Beware polypharmacy.** Sometimes we prescribe combinations of medications more to deal with our own anxieties about a difficult case rather than responding to evidence-based guidelines. Try to clarify the rationale for the medication regimen and document your thinking.
- **Microdosing.** Some patients respond best to very tiny doses of medication (eg, as little as a milligram of an SSRI). This is worth trying in patients who are unable to tolerate higher doses.
- **Megadosing.** Some patients seem to require higher-than-usual doses of medications. If you embark on a high-dose regimen, look for supporting literature (research, case studies), take great care and time in the process, and keep clear documentation.
- **Physiological follow-up.** Be scrupulous about monitoring for potential side effects. Depending on the drug, this may include tracking growth, vital signs, indicated labs, neurological checks (eg, AIMS for patients on antipsychotics), ECGs, etc. Often we assume that the patient's primary care provider will keep up with these tests. Do not count on that. Our patients are less likely to have good primary and preventative care overall, much less good follow-up for the effects of our prescriptions. Check the appendices for some helpful resources.
- **Don't skimp on follow-up.** Patients and their families often have seemingly compelling reasons for avoiding follow-up visits. Push back a little. Soccer practice is important, but medical care is more important. See college kids as often as you would any patient that age, or arrange for them to receive care near their campus.
- **Rating scales.** While we do not discuss rating scales in this book, they can often be helpful in tracking severity of symptoms.
- **Stay patient, thoughtful, and steady.** Families may be tempted to quit medication trials too soon, but we need to remind them that medications take time to work, and that side effects can be alleviated by medication adjustments.

QUICK REVIEW OF DEVELOPMENTAL ASSESSMENT AND PSYCHOPHARMACOLOGY

Infants and young children

- **Assess young children through their interactions.** Young children often demonstrate their functional abilities and challenges best through their interactions with parents and caregivers, not isolated by themselves in your office. Instead, observe them with their caregivers. It is also helpful to observe children in other settings (by video if needed) such as at the home, preschool, park, etc. Early childhood mental health is a subfield of its own, and if you aren't specifically trained or experienced in this field, you deserve support from colleagues.
- **Pharmacodynamic and pharmacokinetic processes in infants.** Drug metabolism and brain effects change from neonate to infant to child to adolescent. Infants and younger children have reduced absorption, plasma protein binding, hepatic metabolism, and both renal and gastrointestinal (pancreatic-mediated) excretion. Higher brain-to-body weight and immaturity of brain development can also play a role in the efficacy of psychotropic medications. CYP metabolism is at about 50%–70% of adult levels in this age group. For any specific medication, dosing may at times require higher or lower mg/kg than for adults. Common examples include stimulants' relative lack of efficacy and increase in frequency of side effects, and the significantly higher toxicity of valproic acid in very young children. For any use of psychotropic medications in young children, it is important to double-check dosing guidelines specific to this population.

School-aged children

- **School-aged kids may need to stay in the waiting room while you have frank discussions with parents.** Parents need to tell you what their children are doing, and yet when this is done in front of the child, it is often experienced as humiliating. Try to have the bulk of such talks out of earshot of the child. You need a safe setting for the child to do this, but it is well worth the effort.
- **School-aged kids often have trouble talking.** School-aged kids may not be able to talk directly about their issues. Instead, their symptoms may become apparent during games, drawing, or other activities. Observation may reveal symptoms such as inattentiveness, trouble reading, expecting defeat, etc. While we do try to talk with children about symptoms, it's not unusual for them to be unable to do so, and this does not need to hamper us. Collateral data from parents, teachers, and others are essential.
- **Be concrete with school-aged children.** They may not report specific difficulties unless you ask them explicitly and use words they understand. They may be very suggestible as well, so yes-no type questions may require follow-up. "How tired are you? A little? A lot? Is it making things different for you?"

- **Liver.** CYP metabolism, while low in early childhood, may be higher than adult levels in middle childhood and may result in a need for higher doses than expected. As always, start low and go slow. Hepatic efficiency typically falls to adult levels with puberty, so some medication doses may need to be reduced, both to alleviate side effects and to use the lowest effective dose.
- **SSRI side effects.** There may be relatively high rates of behavioral activation with SSRIs, with many proposed mechanisms including serotonergic differences in children.
- **Hormones.** We often attribute some of the difficulties of tweens and teens to pubertal changes in hormones and the accompanying social and psychological shifts. It's true. Don't try to medicate normal developmental changes—instead, encourage parents to manage these changes via empathic developmental and behavioral strategies.

Teens

- **Teens often do worse when we leave them in the waiting room.** Managing appointments can become a round robin of seeing the parent and child together, the child alone, the parent alone, etc. Teens often do not do well if we leave them in the waiting room while we talk to parents. They expect and require more confidentiality and ownership of the doctor-patient relationship. Sitting in the waiting room, they are left stewing, possibly making assumptions about what is being discussed. In such cases, try to get your updates from parents via phone calls or email, rather than checking in during the teen's appointment.
- **Teens are not quite young adults.** Teens often have an entirely different manner of processing information and assessing risk than adults. Do not let their adult appearance lead you to presume they can competently weigh the risks and benefits of treatments, and of daily decisions. As a rule, teens will minimize risks. They also tend to prefer being out in the world rather than showing up as planned for appointments. Meanwhile, those who actually *want* to come to see us may well be suffering more severely than they let on.
- **Adult-ish dosing.** Physiologically speaking, most teens can use doses that we typically use in adults.
- **Teens often miss medication.** Teens often miss doses of their medication, and many may be using other substances concurrently. It is important to acknowledge and normalize these behaviors to reduce shame. Ask teens directly whether they have missed medications and whether they have tried any other substances lately. Sometimes medications with longer half-lives (eg, fluoxetine) make sense in order to minimize the effects of missed doses.
- **Supervision and diversion.** More than any other intervention, good supervision is important in the overall plan for teens. While many become able to manage their own medication (and should be taught medication management before going off to college), most need parental guidance and often parental doling out of daily or weekly doses. Keeping parents involved also reduces drug diversion, as long as parents themselves are not using the medications. Close parental monitoring of medication is especially important for teens who are overdose risks.

CLOSING THOUGHT: DON'T DO THIS ALONE

Prescribing for children is challenging. You can't think of everything, and it is important to have access to trusted colleagues and to be part of an ongoing process of case discussion and mutual support. Our field is constantly changing, and the best way to stay on top of the changes is to be engaged in a continual conversation about what we do and how we do it.

ADHD Medications

Generally, in treating kids with ADHD, you should start with psychostimulants, since they are the most effective options. Second-line agents include atomoxetine, bupropion, and alpha agonists.

STIMULANT RECOMMENDATIONS

When choosing a stimulant, the first decision is between an amphetamine or methylphenidate preparation. Methylphenidates are often the go-to as they tend to be more easily tolerated and are as effective as amphetamines for most patients. The second decision is choosing between a long-acting or short-acting stimulant.

For kids who don't like swallowing pills, there are various options. Some long-acting stimulants can be opened and sprinkled on food. There are also short- and long-acting liquid, chewable, and disintegrating brand-name options—though they are expensive and often require pre-authorization. Finally, another option for the pill-phobics is the Daytrana patch.

The case for long-acting stimulants

- More practical: It's easier to take a single dose that lasts through the duration of a school day.
- Addresses acute tachyphylaxis: Response to stimulants diminishes rapidly, but most newer long-acting stimulants release an increasing amount of drug over the 6–12 hour course of the dose, which most people need for the medication to be effective. This avoids the need for multiple short-acting dosage bursts to maintain continued response.
- Decreased stimulant rebound: People sensitive to rebound irritability or worsening of ADHD symptoms often report a more attenuated rebound with long-acting stimulants.

The case for short-acting stimulants

- For situations where a child only requires a few hours of effect, such as a half day of school, an afternoon of completing homework, or a weekend activity.
- Minimizes appetite suppression during meals.
- May be less likely to interfere with sleep.

DOSE EQUIVALENTS

Some kids may need to try different stimulants, or stimulant formulations, before settling on the one that works best for them. The dose equivalents are, luckily, fairly easy to remember.

1. **From amphetamine to another amphetamine**
   - With the exception of Vyvanse, all amphetamines, including Adderall IR and XR, are roughly equivalent in potency. For example, if a child is taking Dexedrine 10 mg TID, you can switch this to Adderall 15 BID or Adderall XR 30 mg QD. That said, some people believe that Dexedrine, being 100% dextroamphetamine, might be more potent than Adderall, which is 75% d-amphetamine and 25% l-amphetamine (eg, Dexedrine 30 mg/day may be closer to 40 mg/day of Adderall). In reality, the effect is likely negligible in most people.
   - Vyvanse is composed of both lysine and amphetamine, with amphetamine making up only about 30% of Vyvanse. This means that it's much less potent than straight Dexedrine. So when switching from another amphetamine to Vyvanse, you have to at least *double the dose,* and sometimes more.

2. **From methylphenidate to another methylphenidate**
   - With the exception of Concerta and Focalin, all methylphenidate preparations are roughly equivalent in potency.
   - Concerta, because of its complex delivery system, delivers less methylphenidate than implied by the mg amount you prescribe. The usual conversion percentage used is 83%, meaning that the body sees 83% of Concerta in methylphenidate equivalents. Thus, Concerta 18 mg is equivalent to methylphenidate 15 mg, 36 mg is equivalent to 30 mg, and so on.
   - Focalin is the dextro-isomer of methylphenidate, which is twice as potent as methylphenidate. Thus, use about half the dose when using Focalin.

3. **From methylphenidate to an amphetamine (or vice versa)**
   - Methylphenidate is roughly half as potent as amphetamine, so Ritalin 10 mg = Dexedrine 5 mg, etc. Consistent with this equivalency, child psychiatrists often dose methylphenidate at 1 mg/kg, whereas they dose amphetamine at 0.5 mg/kg. Conversely, if you're switching from Dexedrine to Ritalin, you would need to double the dosage.

HOW TO SWITCH

Once you've determined the dose equivalence, the actual switching is easy. Don't cross-taper; just have your patient take the last dose of stimulant A on day 1 and start stimulant B on day 2. To be prudent, start the new stimulant at a somewhat lower dose than the calculation you arrived at via the equivalent dose guideline. Those equivalencies are based on averages and may not apply to a given individual.

NON-STIMULANT RECOMMENDATIONS

Although its efficacy cannot compare to stimulants, atomoxetine may be an appropriate first step when you're concerned about diversion or substance misuse. For children with severe tic disorders, guanfacine and clonidine may be indicated with the added benefit of targeting the tics. Alpha agonists are also helpful for addressing the frequent sleep difficulties found in children with ADHD. Patients with comorbid depression or tobacco use may benefit from bupropion. Regardless of your choice, the robust and rapid response frequently seen with stimulants should not be expected with non-stimulant options.

Lastly, some studies have demonstrated small improvements in ADHD symptoms with higher doses of omega-3, specifically eicosapentaenoic acid (EPA), as a supplement; however, this has not been consistently supported in meta-analyses. Limited evidence also exists for gingko biloba in reducing ADHD symptoms. While these should not replace the use of a stimulant or non-stimulant medication, they may be useful as an adjunct and for families who are resistant to medications.

STIMULANT SIDE EFFECTS AND CLASS WARNINGS

- The most common side effects include appetite suppression and insomnia. With long-term use, due to chronic appetite suppression and acute growth hormone inhibition, some literature has reported an average of 0.5 inch decrease in expected height, while several studies have not found significant differences with longer-term follow-up or "drug holidays." Despite this, drug holidays are still useful on weekends and school breaks for patients who struggle with appropriate weight gain, assuming their behavioral functioning remains manageable without medication. Additionally, stimulants should be avoided in patients with anorexia nervosa given their GI side effects.
- Stimulants have been known to unmask underlying tics, and at times they can exacerbate an established Tourette's or tic disorder. To complicate matters further, most children present for ADHD treatment during the age range when tics begin to manifest and worsen. For patients with more severe tics, alpha agonists are worth considering prior to a stimulant trial.
- In patients with a seizure disorder, stimulants may potentially lower the seizure threshold, although the current data are contradictory.
- In patients with a genetic predisposition or history of psychosis, stimulants can potentially exacerbate symptoms in a dose-dependent fashion.
- Patients with comorbid anxiety disorder may experience a worsening of anxiety symptoms.
- Some patients have been known to have increased skin picking, hair pulling, and nail biting behaviors with stimulant medications. Alpha agonists may be helpful here too.
- A few patients may experience an increase in aggressive behaviors or other adverse psychiatric effects (hallucinations, delusions, mania).
- Stimulants may increase heart rate and blood pressure, particularly in older patients; thus, vitals should be monitored at baseline and with subsequent dose adjustments. Patients with cardiovascular symptoms, with a family history of early cardiac death or cardiac arrhythmias, or who are adopted with unknown family histories would benefit from additional consultation from their primary care physician or cardiologist.
- Black box warnings for abuse and dependence: Patients with a history of recent substance use should be followed more closely if stimulants are considered, given the risk of diversion, overuse, and dependence of these medications. Vyvanse is thought to have decreased abuse potential due to being a prodrug that becomes active only after oral ingestion and P450 metabolism.

TABLE 1: ADHD Medications

Brand Name (Generic Name, if different than heading) Year FDA Approved [G] denotes generic availability	Available Strengths (mg except where noted)	Usual Pediatric Dosage Range (starting–max) (mg)	Duration of Action (hours)	Can It Be Split?	Ages Approved for ADHD	Delivery System/Notes (IR = immediate release, CR = controlled release, DR = delayed release, ER = extended release)
Methylphenidates						
Short-acting						
Focalin [G] (Dexmethylphenidate) 2001	2.5, 5, 10	2.5 BID–10 BID	3–4	Yes (not scored)	6–17	Tablet; D-enantiomer of Ritalin; 2x more potent than methylphenidate
Methylin CT [G] 2003	2.5, 5, 10	2.5 BID–20 TID	3–4	Yes	6–17, adults	Chewable, grape-flavored tablet
Methylin oral solution [G] 2002	5 mg/5 mL, 10 mg/5 mL	2.5 BID–20 TID	3–4	NA	6–17, adults	Clear, grape-flavored liquid
Ritalin [G] 1955	5, 10, 20	2.5 BID–20 TID	3–4	Yes	6–17, adults	IR tablet
Intermediate-acting						
Metadate ER [G] Branded generic of Ritalin SR 1999	20	10 QAM–30 BID (max 60/day)	6–8	No	6–17, adults	CR tablet (less predictable because of wax matrix)
Methylin ER [G] Branded generic of Ritalin SR 2000	10, 20	20 QAM–60 QAM	4–8	No	6–17, adults	Hydrophilic polymer tablet; possibly more continuous than others in category
Ritalin SR [G] 1982	10, 20	10 QAM–60 QAM	4–8	No	6–17, adults	CR tablet (less predictable because of wax matrix)
Long-acting						
Aptensio XR 2015	10, 15, 20, 30, 40, 50, 60	10 QAM–60 QAM	8–12	Can be sprinkled; do not crush or chew	6–17, adults	Capsule of 40% IR beads & 60% DR beads
Concerta [G] 2000	18, 27, 36, 54	18 QAM–72 QAM	10–16	No	6–17, adults	CR tablet with 22% IR & 78% DR
Cotempla XR-ODT 2017	8.6, 17.3, 25.9	17.3 QAM–51.8 QAM	8–12	No	6–17	Orally disintegrating, ER with 25% IR & 75% ER
Daytrana patch (Methylphenidate transdermal system) 2006	10, 15, 20, 30	10 QAM–30 QAM Remove after 9 hours	8–12	No	6–17, adults	CR patch; duration can be shortened by decreasing wear time; drug effects may persist for 5 hours after removal
Focalin XR [G] (Dexmethylphenidate XR) 2005	5, 10, 15, 20, 25, 30, 35, 40	5 QAM–30 QAM	8–12	Can be sprinkled; do not crush or chew	6–17, adults	Capsule of 50% IR beads & 50% DR beads; mimics BID dosing; 2x more potent than methylphenidate
Jornay PM 2018	20, 40, 60, 80, 100	20 QPM–100 QPM	8–12; after 10 hour delay in onset	Can be sprinkled; do not crush or chew	6–17, adults	ER capsule of DR beads; taken in evening between 6:30–9:30 pm

Brand Name (Generic Name, if different than heading) Year FDA Approved [G] denotes generic availability	Available Strengths (mg except where noted)	Usual Pediatric Dosage Range (starting–max) (mg)	Duration of Action (hours)	Can It Be Split?	Ages Approved for ADHD	Delivery System/Notes (IR = immediate release, CR = controlled release, DR = delayed release, ER = extended release)
Metadate CD [G] 2001	10, 20, 30, 40, 50, 60	20 QAM–60 QAM	8–12	Can be sprinkled; do not crush or chew	6–17, adults	Capsule of 30% IR beads & 70% DR beads; mimics BID dosing
Quillichew ER 2015	20, 30, 40	20 QAM–60 QAM	8–12	Yes	6–17, adults	Chewable ER for those who will not swallow pills or take liquid; 30% IR & 70% ER
Quillivant XR 2012	25/5 mL	20 QAM–60 QAM	8–12	No	6–17, adults	20% IR & 80% ER in oral solution; shake prior to use
Ritalin LA [G] 2002	10, 20, 30, 40, 60	20 QAM–60 QAM	8–12	Can be sprinkled; do not crush or chew	6–17, adults	Capsule of 50% IR beads & 50% DR beads
Amphetamines						
Short-acting						
Desoxyn [G] (Methamphetamine) 1943	5	5 QAM–10 BID	3–5	Yes	6–17	Tablet
Dexedrine [G] (Dextroamphetamine) 1976	5, 10	3–5 yrs: 2.5 QAM–20 BID; 6–16 yrs: 5 QAM–20 BID	3–5	Yes	3–16	Scored tablet
Evekeo (Amphetamine) 2012	5, 10	3–5 yrs: 2.5 QAM–20 BID; 6–17 yrs: 5 QAM–20 BID	3–5	Yes	3–17	Scored tablet
ProCentra [G] (Dextroamphetamine oral solution) 2008	5 mg/5 mL	5 BID–20 BID	3–5	NA	3–16	Bubblegum-flavored liquid
Zenzedi (Dextroamphetamine) 2013	2.5, 5, 7.5, 10, 15, 20, 30	3–5 yrs: 2.5 BID–20 BID; 6–16 yrs: 5 QAM–20 BID (same as Dexedrine dosing)	3–5	Yes	3–16	Tablet; 5 mg scored, 10 mg double scored, rest unscored
Intermediate-acting						
Adderall [G] (Mixed amphetamine salts) 1960	5, 7.5, 10, 12.5, 15, 20, 30	3–5 yrs: 2.5 QAM–20 BID; 6–17 yrs: 5 QAM–20 BID	6–8	Can be crushed	3–17, adults	Tablet; mixed salt of l- and d-amphetamine
Long-acting						
Adderall XR [G] (Mixed amphetamine salts) 2001	5, 10, 15, 20, 25, 30	6–12 yrs: 5 QAM–30 QAM; 13–17 yrs: 10 QAM–40 QAM	8–12	Can be sprinkled; do not crush or chew	6–17, adults	Capsule of 50% IR beads & 50% DR beads; mixed salt of l- and d-amphetamine; mimics BID dosing
Adzenys XR-ODT (Amphetamine) 2016	3.1, 6.3, 9.4, 12.5, 15.7, 18.8	6–12 yrs: 6.3 QAM–18.8 QAM; 13–17 yrs: 6.3 QAM–12.5 QAM	8–12	No (ODT)	6–17, adults	ER orally disintegrating tablets; 3.1 mg is equivalent to 5 mg mixed salts product; increasing dose preparations are equivalent to 10 mg, 15 mg, 20 mg, 25 mg, and 30 mg respectively

ADHD Medications

Brand Name (Generic Name, if different than heading) Year FDA Approved [G] denotes generic availability	Available Strengths (mg except where noted)	Usual Pediatric Dosage Range (starting–max) (mg)	Duration of Action (hours)	Can It Be Split?	Ages Approved for ADHD	Delivery System/Notes (IR = immediate release, CR = controlled release, DR = delayed release, ER = extended release)
Dexedrine Spansules [G] (Dextroamphetamine) 1976	5, 10, 15	5 QAM–20 BID	6–8	Can be sprinkled; do not crush or chew	3–16	Capsule of 50% IR & 50% sustained release beads
Dyanavel XR (Amphetamine) 2015	2.5 mg/mL	2.5 QAM–20 QAM	8–12	No (oral suspension)	6–17	ER oral suspension allowing once-daily dosing (must shake well); 2.5 mg = 4 mg mixed amphetamine salts
Mydayis (Mixed amphetamine salts) 2017	12.5, 25, 37.5, 50	12.5 QAM–25 QAM	10–12+	Can be sprinkled; do not crush or chew	13–17, adults	pH-dependent ER capsule formulation; may have effect up to 16 hours
Vyvanse (Lisdexamfetamine) 2007	10, 20, 30, 40, 50, 60, 70	30 QAM–70 QAM	8–12	Can be dissolved in water	6–17, adults	Capsule; chewable tablets also available; lisdexamfetamine is prodrug of dextroamphetamine
Non-stimulants						
Intuniv [G] (Guanfacine ER) 2009	1, 2, 3, 4	1–4 QD (do not increase faster than 1 mg/wk) (adolescents 7 mg/day max)	24	No	6–17	ER tablet; do not stop abruptly (rebound hypertension); not a 1:1 conversion from IR; do not give with high-fat meals
Kapvay [G] (Clonidine XR) [G] 2009	0.1, 0.2	0.1 QHS; increase by 0.1 mg/day weekly and give divided BID; max 0.4 QD	12–16	No	6–17	ER tablet; titrate gradually (orthostatic hypotension); avoid abrupt discontinuation; somnolence
Provigil [G] (Modafinil) 1998	100, 200	100 QAM–400 QAM	18–24	Yes (200 mg tabs are scored)	Not FDA-approved for ADHD	Tablet; studies have shown modafinil to be helpful for ADHD, but low incidence of serious rash; minimal data in children
Strattera [G] (Atomoxetine) 2002	10, 18, 25, 40, 60, 80, 100	Dosage varies. See footnote 1 below.	24	No	6–17, adults	Capsule; norepinephrine reuptake inhibitor
Tenex [G] (Guanfacine IR) 1986	1, 2	1–4 QD (do not increase faster than 1 mg/wk)	17	Can be crushed	Not FDA-approved for kids or ADHD, approved only for adults 18+ for hypertension	Tablet
Wellbutrin [G] (Bupropion) 1985	75, 100	1.4–6 mg/kg/day	6–9	Yes	Not FDA-approved for ADHD	Tablet; bupropion SR & XL versions exist

[1] Strattera dosing: Weight <70 kg, start 0.5 mg/kg, target 1.2 mg/kg, max 1.4 mg/kg; weight >70 kg, 40–100 mg

AMPHETAMINE (Adzenys XR-ODT, Dyanavel XR, Evekeo) Fact Sheet

PEDIATRIC FDA INDICATIONS:
ADHD (Adzenys XR-ODT and Dyanavel XR: children >6; Evekeo: children >3).

ADULT FDA INDICATIONS:
ADHD (Adzenys XR-ODT); narcolepsy (Evekeo); obesity (Evekeo).

OFF-LABEL USES:
Treatment-resistant depression.

DOSAGE FORMS:
Tablets (Evekeo): 5 mg, 10 mg (scored).
ER orally disintegrating tablets (Adzenys XR-ODT): 3.1 mg, 6.3 mg, 9.4 mg, 12.5 mg, 15.7 mg, 18.8 mg.
ER oral suspension (Dyanavel XR): 2.5 mg/mL.

PEDIATRIC DOSAGE GUIDANCE:
- Tablets (Evekeo):
  – Children 3–5: Start 2.5 mg QAM, increase in 2.5 mg/day increments weekly to maximum of 40 mg/day in divided doses.
  – Children 6–17: Start 5 mg QAM, increase in 5 mg/day increments weekly to maximum of 40 mg/day in divided doses.
- ER ODT (Adzenys XR-ODT):
  – Start 6.3 mg QAM, increase in 3.1–6.3 mg/day increments weekly. Maximum of 18.8 mg/day (ages 6–12) or 12.5 mg/day (ages 13–17).
- ER oral suspension (Dyanavel XR):
  – Start 2.5 mg–5 mg QAM, increase in 2.5–10 mg/day increments every 4–7 days. Maximum 20 mg/day.

MONITORING: Weight, height, BP/P; ECG.

COST: $$$$

SIDE EFFECTS:
- Most common: abdominal pain, decreased appetite, weight loss, insomnia, headache, nervousness.
- Serious but rare: See class warnings in chapter introduction.

MECHANISM, PHARMACOKINETICS, AND DRUG INTERACTIONS:
- Stimulant that inhibits reuptake of dopamine and norepinephrine.
- Metabolized primarily via CYP2D6; t ½: 11 hours.
- Avoid use with MAOIs, antacids.

EVIDENCE AND CLINICAL PEARLS:
- FDA-approved, many studies, history of clinical efficacy and safety, & larger effect size than non-stimulants.
- Racemic l-isomer is more potent than d-isomer in peripheral activity (more cardiovascular effects, tics).
- There may be less appetite suppressant effects with racemic mixture compared to dextroamphetamine.
- Divide IR (Evekeo) doses by 4–6 hour intervals.
- Approximate equivalence doses of Adzenys XR-ODT and mixed amphetamine salts XR (Adderall XR) are: 3.1 mg = 5 mg, 6.3 mg = 10 mg, 9.4 mg = 15 mg, 12.5 mg = 20 mg, 15.7 mg = 25 mg, 18.8 mg = 30 mg.
- Shake Dyanavel XR oral suspension for extended release. 2.5 mg/mL = 4 mg of mixed amphetamine salts.
- Amphetamines are not interchangeable on a mg:mg basis. When switching, use a lowered dose and adjust.

FUN FACT:
The term "amphetamine" is the contracted form of the chemical "alpha-methylphenethylamine." Its first pharmacologic use was when pharmaceutical company Smith, Kline and French sold amphetamine under the trade name Benzedrine as a decongestant inhaler.

BOTTOM LINE:
Newer formulations of an old drug come with a high price tag. Stick to the usual amphetamine products like mixed amphetamine salts unless liquid or ODT dosing is absolutely necessary.

ATOMOXETINE (Strattera) Fact Sheet [G]

PEDIATRIC FDA INDICATIONS:
ADHD (6–17 years).

ADULT FDA INDICATIONS:
ADHD.

OFF-LABEL USES:
Treatment-resistant depression.

DOSAGE FORMS:
Capsules (G): 10 mg, 18 mg, 25 mg, 40 mg, 60 mg, 80 mg, 100 mg.

PEDIATRIC DOSAGE GUIDANCE:
- Children >70 kg: Start 40 mg QAM for 3 days, ↑ to 80 mg QAM, may ↑ to 100 mg/day after 2–4 weeks if needed (max 100 mg/day); may divide doses >40 mg/day (divided dosing in morning and late afternoon/early evening).
- Children <70 kg: Start 0.5 mg/kg QAM for 3 days, ↑ to 1.2 mg/kg QAM, may ↑ to max 1.4 mg/kg/day or 100 mg/day (whichever is less) after 2–4 weeks, if needed; may divide doses >0.5 mg/kg/day (divided dosing in morning and late afternoon/early evening).

MONITORING: BP/P, LFTs.

COST: $$$

SIDE EFFECTS:
- Most common: headache, abdominal pain, decreased appetite, fatigue, nausea, vomiting.
- Serious but rare: Class warning for suicidal ideation in children and teens. Severe hepatic injury including increased hepatic enzymes (up to 40 times normal) and jaundice (bilirubin up to 12 times upper limit of normal). Increased blood pressure (↑ 15–20 mmHg) and heart rate (↑ 20 bpm).

MECHANISM, PHARMACOKINETICS, AND DRUG INTERACTIONS:
- Selective norepinephrine reuptake inhibitor (NRI).
- Metabolized primarily via CYP2D6; t ½: 5 hours.
- Avoid use with MAOIs. Exercise caution with 2D6 inhibitors such as fluoxetine, paroxetine, and quinidine (increased atomoxetine serum levels); use slower titration and do not exceed 80 mg/day in presence of 2D6 inhibitors or in 2D6 poor metabolizers.

EVIDENCE AND CLINICAL PEARLS:
- Effective and FDA-approved for ADHD; however, several studies clearly show it does not produce as robust of a treatment effect as stimulants.
- QAM dosing is as effective as BID, but BID dosing has better GI tolerability. Can also be dosed at bedtime if it causes fatigue.
- Appears to be more effective in improving attention than in controlling hyperactivity.

FUN FACT:
Atomoxetine was originally known as "tomoxetine"; however, the FDA requested that the name be changed because the similarity to "tamoxifen" could lead to dispensing errors.

BOTTOM LINE:
Advantages: Unlike stimulants, atomoxetine has no abuse potential, causes less insomnia and anxiety, and is unlikely to worsen tics.

Disadvantages: It is generally less effective than stimulants, and takes longer to work (2–4 weeks).

CLONIDINE (Catapres, Kapvay) Fact Sheet [G]

PEDIATRIC FDA INDICATIONS:
ADHD (6–17 years [ER formulation only]).

ADULT FDA INDICATIONS:
Hypertension.

OFF-LABEL USES:
ADHD (IR); insomnia; anxiety; PTSD; opioid withdrawal; ASD; ODD; Tourette's.

DOSAGE FORMS:
- IR tablets (**Catapres, G**): 0.1 mg, 0.2 mg, 0.3 mg.
- ER tablets (**Kapvay, G**): 0.1 mg, 0.2 mg.

PEDIATRIC DOSAGE GUIDANCE:
- ADHD or anxiety:
  - ER: 0.1 QHS; increase by 0.1 mg/day weekly and give divided BID; max 0.4 QD
  - IR: 0.05 mg QHS; increase by 0.05 mg/day increments every 3–7 days; max 0.2 mg/day for 27–40.5 kg, 0.3 mg/day for 40.5–45 kg, or 0.4 mg/day for >45 kg; doses may be divided up to QID dosing
- Insomnia: Start 0.05 mg IR QHS, titrate if needed by 0.05 mg (<45 kg) or 0.1 mg (>45 kg) increments every 3–7 days; max 0.4 mg nightly, though most will respond to doses ≤0.2 mg at bedtime.

MONITORING: BP.

COST: IR: $; ER: $$$

SIDE EFFECTS:
- Most common: somnolence, fatigue, dizziness, headache.
- Serious but rare: hypotension, syncope, orthostasis.

MECHANISM, PHARMACOKINETICS, AND DRUG INTERACTIONS:
- Centrally acting alpha-2 adrenergic agonist.
- Metabolized primary through liver (CYP unknown); t ½: 12–16 hours.
- Avoid use with MAOIs. Additive effects with other antihypertensives.

EVIDENCE AND CLINICAL PEARLS:
- Studies support the use of clonidine to decrease residual hyperactivity, impulsivity, and aggression in ADHD.
- Several small limited (chart reviews, case series, descriptive, or retrospective) studies have supported the efficacy of clonidine as a sleep aid in children with and without ADHD, autism spectrum disorders, developmental delays, and genetic syndromes; however, a small systematic chart review showed significant subjective improvement in sleep in children, but only a nonsignificant trend for improvement of sleep in adolescents.
- Avoid abrupt discontinuation because of potential risk for rebound hypertension.
- Clonidine is a preferred agent for sleep by many child psychiatrists, but little empirical evidence exists to support this use. Still, anecdotal clinical experience suggests clonidine is generally safe and effective for insomnia, particularly in kids with ADHD.
- Generally more sedating than guanfacine.

FUN FACT:
In the early 1960s, Boehringer Ingelheim wished to synthesize a peripherally active adrenergic drug for nasal decongestion as nose drops. After administering the potential compound to a secretary, she fell asleep for 24 hours, developing low blood pressure, low pulse, and dry mouth. This compound was subsequently developed as clonidine for treating hypertension.

BOTTOM LINE:
Clonidine is a good option in kids with ADHD who also have tics, who experience excessive anxiety or insomnia on stimulants, or in whom substance misuse is a concern. Commonly used off label for anxiety and insomnia, but efficacy data are limited.

DEXMETHYLPHENIDATE (Focalin) Fact Sheet [G]

PEDIATRIC FDA INDICATIONS:
ADHD (6–17 years [IR and XR]).

ADULT FDA INDICATIONS:
ADHD (XR only).

OFF-LABEL USES:
Narcolepsy; obesity; treatment-resistant depression.

DOSAGE FORMS:
- **Tablets (G):** 2.5 mg, 5 mg, 10 mg.
- **ER capsules (G):** 5 mg, 10 mg, 15 mg, 20 mg, 25 mg, 30 mg, 35 mg, 40 mg.

PEDIATRIC DOSAGE GUIDANCE:
- IR: Start 2.5 mg BID, ↑ by 5 mg–10 mg/day every 7 days. Max 20 mg/day; divide IR doses by at least 4 hours.
- ER: Start 5 mg QAM, ↑ by 5 mg/day every 7 days. Max 30 mg/day.

MONITORING: Weight, height, BP/P; ECG.

COST: IR: $; ER: $$$

SIDE EFFECTS:
- Most common: decreased appetite, insomnia, anxiety, GI distress, irritability, tics, headache, tachycardia, hypertension, dry mouth.
- Serious but rare: See cardiovascular class warning in chapter introduction.

MECHANISM, PHARMACOKINETICS, AND DRUG INTERACTIONS:
- Stimulant that inhibits reuptake of dopamine and norepinephrine.
- Metabolized primarily via de-esterification, not CYP450; t ½: 2–4.5 hours (2–3 hours in children); ER delivers 50% of dose immediately and 50% about 5 hours later.
- Avoid use with MAOIs.

EVIDENCE AND CLINICAL PEARLS:
- Several randomized controlled trials and meta-analysis have shown dexmethylphenidate, like other stimulants, is effective for ADHD with a large treatment effect size.
- Focalin is the d-isomer of methylphenidate and is 2x more potent than methylphenidate, which is why it is prescribed at about half the dose.
- Use the same total daily dose of Focalin IR as Focalin XR.
- Focalin XR capsules contain 2 kinds of beads: Half are immediate release beads and half are enteric coated delayed release beads. A single, once-daily dose of XR capsule provides the same amount of dexmethylphenidate as 2 IR tablets given 4 hours apart.
- The ER capsules cannot be split in half. However, they can be opened and the beads sprinkled over food. The patient should then eat all that food—eating half won't work to split the dose accurately because it won't be possible to determine if the eaten portion contains more immediate release or delayed release beads.
- Give with food if GI side effects occur.

FUN FACT:
With 2 stereoactive centers, methylphenidate has 4 possible stereoisomers. Of the 4, dexmethylphenidate is the most active biologically.

BOTTOM LINE:
Focalin is just Ritalin but more potent. It's available as a generic and may mean fewer tablets for patients. Focalin XR only recently went generic, so it will likely remain quite expensive for a while.

DEXTROAMPHETAMINE (Dexedrine) Fact Sheet [G]

PEDIATRIC FDA INDICATIONS:
ADHD (3–17 years); **narcolepsy** (6–17 years).

ADULT FDA INDICATIONS:
Narcolepsy.

OFF-LABEL USES:
Obesity; treatment-resistant depression.

DOSAGE FORMS:
- **Tablets (Dexedrine) (G):** 5 mg, 10 mg (scored).
- **Tablets (Zenzedi):** 2.5 mg, 5 mg, 7.5 mg, 10 mg, 15 mg, 20 mg, 30 mg (5 mg scored, 10 mg double scored; rest unscored).
- **ER capsules (Dexedrine Spansules) (G):** 5 mg, 10 mg, 15 mg.
- **Liquid (ProCentra) (G):** 5 mg/5 mL.

PEDIATRIC DOSAGE GUIDANCE:
- ADHD (IR and ER):
  - Children >6 years: Start 5 mg QAM; ↑ by 5 mg/day at weekly intervals to max 60 mg/day, though doses >40 mg/day rarely more effective. Divide IR dose QD–TID.
  - Children 3–5 years: Start 2.5 mg QAM; ↑ by 2.5 mg/day weekly to max 60 mg/day, though doses >40 mg/day rarely more effective. Divide IR dose QD–TID.
- Narcolepsy (IR and ER):
  - Start 5 mg QAM (ages 6–11) or 10 mg QAM (ages 12–17); ↑ by 5 mg/day (ages 6–11) or 10 mg/day (ages 12–17) weekly to max 60 mg/day. Divide IR dose QD–TID.

MONITORING: Weight, height, BP/P; ECG.

COST: IR: $$ (ProCentra: $$$$); ER: $$$

SIDE EFFECTS:
- Most common: abdominal pain, anorexia, nausea, tics, insomnia, tachycardia, and headache.
- Serious but rare: See class warnings in chapter introduction.

MECHANISM, PHARMACOKINETICS, AND DRUG INTERACTIONS:
- Stimulant that inhibits reuptake of dopamine and norepinephrine.
- Metabolized primarily through CYP450 2D6 (minor) and glucuronidation; t ½: 12 hours.
- Avoid use with MAOIs, antacids.

EVIDENCE AND CLINICAL PEARLS:
- At least 5 randomized clinical trials, some dating back to the 1970s, support the efficacy of dextroamphetamine in children with ADHD.
- Dextroamphetamine is the more potent d-isomer of amphetamine; it has potentially less peripheral effects (eg, motor tics) than racemic mix (eg, mixed amphetamine salts like Adderall, amphetamine, or methamphetamine).
- Doses of IR tablets and oral solution can be given at intervals of 4–6 hours.
- Dextroamphetamine is the only stimulant, other than Adderall IR, approved for children <6 years (approved for children >3 years).
- The newer Zenzedi brand offers more dosing flexibility options, but is more expensive than generic IR tablets.
- Also available as D,L racemic mixture of amphetamine as Evekeo tablets, Adzenys XR-ODT, and Dyanavel XR oral suspension (see amphetamine fact sheet).

FUN FACT:
Dexys Midnight Runners, the British band famous for its song "Come On Eileen" (1982), derived their name from Dexedrine—"Dexys" after the drug's name and "Midnight Runners" in reference to the energy it provides.

BOTTOM LINE:
Good drug, with very long history of experience, available in short- and long-acting formulations as generics.

GUANFACINE (Intuniv, Tenex) Fact Sheet [G]

PEDIATRIC FDA INDICATIONS:
ADHD (6–17 years [ER formulation only]), as monotherapy or adjunctive therapy to stimulants.

ADULT FDA INDICATIONS:
Hypertension.

OFF-LABEL USES:
Conduct disorder; Tourette's and motor tics; agitation in autism spectrum disorder; migraine prophylaxis; opioid withdrawal; anxiety and PTSD; insomnia.

DOSAGE FORMS:
- **IR tablets (Tenex, G):** 1 mg, 2 mg.
- **ER tablets (Intuniv, G):** 1 mg, 2 mg, 3 mg, 4 mg.

PEDIATRIC DOSAGE GUIDANCE:
- ADHD or anxiety:
  – IR dosing depends on weight.
    ○ 27–40.5 kg (55–90 lbs): Start 0.5 mg QHS, ↑ by 0.5 mg/day at weekly intervals up to 1.5 mg/day; may ↑ to 2 mg/day after 2 weeks; max 2 mg/day in 2–4 divided doses.
    ○ 40.5–45 kg (90–99 lbs): Start 0.5 mg QHS, ↑ by 0.5 mg/day at weekly intervals; max 1 mg per dose, 3 mg/day.
    ○ >45 kg (>99 lbs): Start 1 mg QHS, ↑ by 1 mg/day at weekly intervals up to 3 mg/day; may ↑ to 4 mg/day after 2 weeks; max 1 mg per dose, 4 mg/day.
  – ER: Start 1 mg QHS, ↑ by 1 mg/day at weekly intervals; max 4 mg/day. Alternative: 0.05 mg/kg–0.12 mg/kg QD or QHS; max 4 mg/day. Doses up to 7 mg/day ER studied as monotherapy in adolescents.
- Insomnia: Use IR: start low, go slow, typically 0.5 mg QHS, increasing by 0.5 mg/day at weekly intervals; max 3 mg/day.

MONITORING: BP.

COST: IR: $; ER: $

SIDE EFFECTS:
- Most common: dry mouth, somnolence, dizziness, constipation, fatigue, headache.
- Serious but rare: hypotension, syncope, orthostasis.

MECHANISM, PHARMACOKINETICS, AND DRUG INTERACTIONS:
- Centrally acting, selective alpha-2 adrenergic agonist.
- Metabolized primarily through CYP3A4; t ½: 13–14 hours in children (16–18 hours in adults).
- Avoid use with MAOIs. Caution with 3A4 inhibitors (eg, clarithromycin, fluvoxamine) and inducers (eg, St. John's wort, carbamazepine).

EVIDENCE AND CLINICAL PEARLS:
- At least 6 randomized placebo-controlled trials and a meta-analysis show efficacy in children with ADHD.
- Pilot study of 83 children with GAD, separation anxiety, or social anxiety found guanfacine treatment resulted in greater subjective improvement of anxiety than placebo, but no improvement on other measures of anxiety.
- One negative randomized trial for insomnia in children with ADHD found decreased total sleep time of nearly an hour, with kids taking more time to fall asleep.
- Guanfacine IR and ER are not interchangeable on a mg:mg basis. When switching, taper and retitrate.
- Guanfacine tends to be less sedating than clonidine, another alpha agonist.
- If a child misses 2 or more consecutive doses, consider repeating titration.
- ER tablets should not be taken with a high-fat meal due to increased medication exposure.
- Minimize side effects, especially somnolence, by administering at bedtime.
- Monitor BP, especially during initial dosing titration.
- There is a risk of nervousness, anxiety, and possibly rebound hypertension 2–4 days after abrupt discontinuation. Taper dose in 1 mg/day decrements, every 3–7 days.

FUN FACT:
Some prescribers have taken advantage of guanfacine's sympatholytic properties for the treatment of anxiety disorders in children as well as nightmares and dissociative symptoms in PTSD.

BOTTOM LINE:
Guanfacine's advantages over stimulants include no worsening of tic disorders, lack of abuse potential, and no insomnia. However, its delayed onset of effect (2–4 weeks) and lower efficacy rates make it a second-line choice for ADHD generally. ER is now available in generic and easier to use than IR. Commonly used off label for anxiety and insomnia, but efficacy data are limited.

LISDEXAMFETAMINE (Vyvanse) Fact Sheet

PEDIATRIC FDA INDICATIONS:
ADHD (6–17 years).

ADULT FDA INDICATIONS:
ADHD; binge eating disorder (BED).

OFF-LABEL USES:
Narcolepsy; obesity; treatment-resistant depression.

DOSAGE FORMS:
- **Capsules:** 10 mg, 20 mg, 30 mg, 40 mg, 50 mg, 60 mg, 70 mg.
- **Chewable tablets:** 10 mg, 20 mg, 30 mg, 40 mg, 50 mg, 60 mg.

PEDIATRIC DOSAGE GUIDANCE:
Start 30 mg QAM, ↑ by 10 mg–20 mg/day at weekly intervals. Target lowest effective dose; max 70 mg/day.

MONITORING: Weight, height, BP/P; ECG.

COST: $$$$

SIDE EFFECTS:
- Most common: insomnia, anorexia, abdominal pain, irritability, agitation, tics, decreased appetite, increased heart rate, jitteriness, anxiety.
- Serious but rare: See class warnings in chapter introduction.

MECHANISM, PHARMACOKINETICS, AND DRUG INTERACTIONS:
- Stimulant that inhibits reuptake of dopamine and norepinephrine.
- Metabolized primarily through non-CYP-mediated hepatic and/or intestinal metabolism; t ½: lisdexamfetamine (inactive prodrug) <1 hour; dextroamphetamine (active metabolite) 12 hours. Dextroamphetamine metabolized by CYP2D6.
- Avoid use with MAOIs and antacids. Caution with antihypertensives (decreased efficacy of antihypertensive). Caution with 2D6 inhibitors, which may increase stimulant effects.

EVIDENCE AND CLINICAL PEARLS:
- At least five randomized controlled trials and a meta-analysis support efficacy of lisdexamfetamine in children with ADHD.
- Lisdexamfetamine is dextroamphetamine with the chemical lysine bound to it, which renders it inactive. It remains inactive until GI enzymes cleave off lysine and convert it to active dextroamphetamine. This means that drug abusers can't get high by snorting it or injecting it.
- Anecdotally, Vyvanse has a more gradual onset and offset than other stimulants, and may cause fewer side effects than other amphetamines.
- Taking with food decreases the effect slightly and delays peak levels by an hour. If patients feel it's not "kicking in" fast enough, have them take it earlier or on an empty stomach.
- Lisdexamfetamine 70 mg is equivalent to 30 mg of mixed amphetamine salts (Adderall).
- While indicated for BED, it is not approved for use as a weight-loss or anti-obesity agent, nor has it been studied in children.

FUN FACT:
The manufacturer of Vyvanse pursued an indication as an add-on medication for depression, but disappointing results in clinical trials put an end to this effort.

BOTTOM LINE:
Vyvanse may have a gentler, "smoother" side effect profile than other amphetamines, and probably has a lower risk of diversion or abuse. However, its high cost means insurance companies don't like to pay for it without prior authorizations.

METHAMPHETAMINE (Desoxyn) Fact Sheet [G]

PEDIATRIC FDA INDICATIONS:
ADHD (6–17 years); **obesity** (12–17 years).

ADULT FDA INDICATIONS:
Obesity.

DOSAGE FORMS:
Tablets (G): 5 mg.

PEDIATRIC DOSAGE GUIDANCE:
ADHD: Start 5 mg QAM–BID, ↑ by 5 mg/day at weekly intervals to max 20 mg/day, divided BID.

MONITORING: Weight, height, BP/P; ECG.

COST: $$$$

SIDE EFFECTS:
- Most common: anorexia, tachycardia, dizziness, insomnia, tremor, tics, restlessness, headache, constipation (decreased GI motility). Dental complications, such as poor dental hygiene, diffuse cavities, bruxism, and tooth wear, may develop with abuse.
- Serious but rare: See class warnings in chapter introduction.

MECHANISM, PHARMACOKINETICS, AND DRUG INTERACTIONS:
- Stimulant that inhibits reuptake of dopamine and norepinephrine.
- Metabolized primarily through CYP2D6 to active metabolite (amphetamine); t ½: 4–5 hours.
- Avoid use with MAOIs and antacids. Caution with 2D6 inhibitors, which may increase stimulant effects.

EVIDENCE AND CLINICAL PEARLS:
- FDA indication, but very limited published data in children.
- High risk of abuse.
- Not widely used (DEA reports that there were only 16,000 prescriptions written in 2012). When prescribed for obesity, the recommendation is for short-term (ie, a few weeks) use only and as an adjunct to caloric restriction due to its high addiction and diversion potential.
- CNS stimulating effect is approximately equal to or greater than that of amphetamine but less than that of dextroamphetamine; less BP elevation than with amphetamine.

FUN FACTS:
Desoxyn is the same as the abused street drug methamphetamine, just pharmaceutical grade. Although methamphetamine and amphetamine were long thought to be available only via laboratories, methamphetamine has been reported to occur naturally in certain acacia trees that grow in West Texas.

BOTTOM LINE:
Highly addictive substance; its use is generally not recommended. Watch the television show *Breaking Bad* if you're not convinced!

METHYLPHENIDATE IR (Ritalin) Fact Sheet [G]

PEDIATRIC FDA INDICATIONS:
ADHD (6–17 years).

ADULT FDA INDICATIONS:
ADHD; narcolepsy.

OFF-LABEL USES:
Obesity; treatment-resistant depression.

DOSAGE FORMS:
- **Tablets (G):** 5 mg, 10 mg, 20 mg.
- **Chewable tablets (G):** 2.5 mg, 5 mg, 10 mg.
- **Oral solution (G):** 5 mg/5 mL, 10 mg/5 mL.

PEDIATRIC DOSAGE GUIDANCE:
- ADHD: Children 6–17 years: Start 0.3 mg/kg BID or 2.5 mg–5 mg BID before breakfast and lunch, increase by 0.1 mg/kg/dose or 5 mg–10 mg/day at weekly intervals to a max of 2 mg/kg/day or 60 mg/day.
- Narcolepsy: same dosing as ADHD.

MONITORING: Weight, height, BP/P; ECG.

COST: $ (chewable tablets and oral solution: $$$)

SIDE EFFECTS:
- Most common: insomnia, headache, nervousness, abdominal pain, nausea, vomiting, anorexia, weight loss, affect lability, tics.
- Serious but rare: See class warnings in chapter introduction.

MECHANISM, PHARMACOKINETICS, AND DRUG INTERACTIONS:
- Stimulant that inhibits reuptake of dopamine and norepinephrine.
- Hepatic metabolism via carboxylesterase CES1A1, not CYP450 isoenzymes; t ½: 2–4 hours.
- Avoid use with MAOIs, antacids.

EVIDENCE AND CLINICAL PEARLS:
- FDA-approved with many studies and long history of clinical use supporting its efficacy and safety, with a larger treatment effect size than non-stimulant medications.
- Methylphenidate generally causes fewer side effects than amphetamine preparations—patients are less likely to report feeling "wired."
- While all stimulants may unmask tics, a Cochrane review of 8 randomized trials showed that methylphenidate did not worsen tics in children with ADHD and a tic disorder; in some cases it even improved tics.
- Methylin chewable tablet: Administer with at least 8 ounces of water or other fluid.

FUN FACT:
Methylphenidate was synthesized by Ciba (now Novartis) chemist Leandro Panizzon. His wife, Marguerite, had low blood pressure and would take the stimulant before playing tennis. He named the substance "Ritaline" (yes, with the "e" on the end) after his wife's nickname, Rita.

BOTTOM LINE:
Better side effect profile and somewhat lower abuse potential than amphetamines. However, patients often prefer the "kick" they get from Adderall.

METHYLPHENIDATE ER (Concerta, Ritalin-SR and LA) Fact Sheet [G]

PEDIATRIC FDA INDICATIONS:
ADHD (6–17 years).

ADULT FDA INDICATIONS:
ADHD; narcolepsy.

OFF-LABEL USES:
Obesity; treatment-resistant depression.

DOSAGE FORMS (MORE COMMONLY USED):
- SR tablets (Ritalin SR, Metadate ER, Methylin ER) (G): 10 mg, 20 mg.
- ER capsules (Ritalin LA) (G): 10 mg, 20 mg, 30 mg, 40 mg, 60 mg (50% IR/50% ER).
- ER capsules (Metadate CD) (G): 10 mg, 20 mg, 30 mg, 40 mg, 50 mg, 60 mg (30% IR/70% ER).
- ER capsules (Aptensio XR): 10 mg, 15 mg, 20 mg, 30 mg, 40 mg, 50 mg, 60 mg (40% IR/60% ER).
- ER capsule osmotic release oral system (OROS) (Concerta) (G): 18 mg, 27 mg, 36 mg, 54 mg (22% IR/78% ER).
- ER oral suspension (Quillivant XR): 25 mg/5 mL (20% IR/80% ER).
- ER chewable tablets (Quillichew ER): 20 mg, 30 mg, 40 mg (30% IR/70% ER).
- ER orally disintegrating tablets (Cotempla): 8.6 mg, 17.3 mg, 25.9 mg (25% IR/75% ER).
- ER capsules (Jornay PM): 20 mg, 40 mg, 60 mg, 80 mg, 100 mg (onset delayed 10 hours).

PEDIATRIC DOSAGE GUIDANCE:
- Intermediate-acting (Ritalin SR, Metadate ER, Methylin ER):
  – Titrate to effective daily dose with IR, then switch to equivalent 8-hour SR or ER dose QAM–BID or start 10 mg QAM and increase by 10 mg/day increments weekly; max 60 mg/day.
- Long-acting (Aptensio XR, Metadate CD, Ritalin LA, Quillivant XR):
  – Start 10 mg–20 mg QAM; ↑ by 10 mg/day at weekly intervals; max 60 mg/day.
- Long-acting (Cotempla):
  – Start 17.3 mg QAM; ↑ by 8.6–17.3 mg/day at weekly intervals; max 51.8 mg/day.
  – 8.6 mg, 17.3 mg, 25.9 mg equivalent to 10 mg, 20 mg, 30 mg of other methylphenidate formulations, respectively.
- Long-acting (Concerta):
  – Start 18 mg QAM (ages 6–12) or 36 mg (ages 13–17) QAM, ↑ by 18 mg/day in weekly intervals to max 54 mg/day (ages 6–12) or 72 mg/day (ages 13–17).
  – If switching from different form of methylphenidate:
    ○ 10 mg–15 mg/day: Use 18 mg QAM.
    ○ 20 mg–30 mg/day: Use 36 mg QAM.
    ○ 30 mg–45 mg/day: Use 54 mg QAM.
    ○ 40 mg–60 mg/day: Use 72 mg QAM.
    ○ 27 mg dose is available for situations in which a dose between 18 mg and 36 mg is desired.
- Jornay PM:
  – Start 20 mg daily in the evening and increase in increments of 20 mg/day up to maximum of 100 mg/day. Adjust timing between 6:30 and 9:30 p.m.

MONITORING: Weight, height, BP/P; ECG.

COST: $$$ (except Aptensio XR, Jornay PM, Quillivant XR, and Quillichew ER: $$$$)

SIDE EFFECTS AND MECHANISM, PHARMACOKINETICS, AND DRUG INTERACTIONS:
See methylphenidate IR fact sheet.

EVIDENCE AND CLINICAL PEARLS:
- FDA-approved with many studies and long history of clinical use supporting its efficacy and safety, with a larger treatment effect size than non-stimulant medications.
- ER capsules contain mixture of 30% IR and 70% ER beads. Aptensio XR, a new branded formulation of ER capsules, contains a mixture of 40% IR and 60% ER beads. Ritalin LA and its generic ER capsules are a combination of 50% IR and 50% DR beads. These products mimic BID dosing of IR. Cotempla delivers a mixture of 25% IR and 75% ER in an orally disintegrating extended release formulation. Jornay PM dosed in evening.
- Concerta is based on the OROS osmotic delivery system (also used for Invega). 22% of the dose is immediate (with effects in 1–2 hours) and 78% is delayed. If you prescribe a generic, you may need to investigate carefully to ensure that the delivery system is an OROS pump system. To avoid insomnia, dosing should be completed by noon.
- ER capsules may be opened and contents sprinkled onto a small amount (1 tablespoon) of cold applesauce (swallow without chewing). Do NOT open, crush, or cut Concerta.

BOTTOM LINE:
There are many longer-acting methylphenidate preparations. Two good options are Concerta and Ritalin LA.

METHYLPHENIDATE TRANSDERMAL (Daytrana) Fact Sheet

PEDIATRIC FDA INDICATIONS:
ADHD (6–17 years).

ADULT FDA INDICATIONS:
ADHD.

DOSAGE FORMS:
Transdermal patch: 10 mg, 15 mg, 20 mg, 30 mg/9 hour.

PEDIATRIC DOSAGE GUIDANCE:
Start 10 mg/9 hour patch QAM (for initial therapy or for patients switching from other methylphenidate preparations, regardless of dose). Apply to hip 2 hours before an effect is needed and remove 9 hours after application (drug effects may persist for 5 hours after removal). Increase dose at weekly intervals by using next higher dose system. May be removed in <9 hours if shorter duration is desired or if late-day side effects occur. Rotate application sites. Max 30 mg QD.

MONITORING: Weight, height, BP/P; ECG.

COST: $$$$

SIDE EFFECTS:
- Most common: headache, insomnia, irritability, decreased appetite, anorexia, nausea, tics, application site reaction (10%–40% incidence in children).
- Serious but rare: allergic contact dermatitis/sensitization, characterized by intense local reactions (eg, edema, papules) that may spread beyond patch site; sensitization may subsequently manifest systemically with other routes of methylphenidate administration.

MECHANISM, PHARMACOKINETICS, AND DRUG INTERACTIONS:
- Stimulant that inhibits reuptake of dopamine and norepinephrine.
- Hepatic metabolism via carboxylesterase CES1A1, not CYP450 isoenzymes; t ½: 3–4 hours.
- Avoid use with MAOIs, antacids.

EVIDENCE AND CLINICAL PEARLS:
- FDA-approved with several studies supporting its efficacy and safety, with a larger treatment effect size than non-stimulant medications, including in preschoolers (albeit no FDA indication for this age group).
- Apply patch to clean, dry area of the hip; don't apply to waistline or to areas under tight clothes, as it may rub off. Alternate sites daily (eg, opposite hip). Absorption not affected by perspiration. Remove after 9 hours. If dislodged, replace with a new patch but remove within the 9-hour total wear time.
- Clinical effect usually seen in 2 hours and lasts approximately 12 hours.
- Exposure of application site to a heat source (eg, hair dryer, heating pad, electric blanket) may increase the amount of drug absorbed.
- In June 2015, the FDA added a warning that Daytrana could cause chemical leukoderma, a permanent loss of skin color. These reactions are irreversible and not harmful but can be disfiguring to patients. Instruct patients to contact their physician if they notice skin color changes or lightening of skin areas; in such cases, an alternative medication should be considered.
- The manufacturer recommends to not cut the patch as it may release too much medication or inconsistently.

FUN FACT:
Since 2006, Shire Pharmaceuticals has issued at least 10 recalls of Daytrana patches because users have had difficulty removing the protective cover from the patch. Recall costs have reached into the millions.

BOTTOM LINE:
Daytrana is helpful for kids who, for whatever reason, cannot use any of the wide variety of oral stimulant preparations. Otherwise, we don't recommend it due to high cost, lag time for onset of effect, and the side effect of rash, which is pretty common and unpleasant.

MIXED AMPHETAMINE SALTS (Adderall) Fact Sheet [G]

PEDIATRIC FDA INDICATIONS:
ADHD (3–17 years for IR, 6–17 years for XR, 13–17 years for Mydayis); **narcolepsy** (6–17 years).

ADULT FDA INDICATIONS:
ADHD; narcolepsy.

OFF-LABEL USES:
Obesity; treatment-resistant depression.

DOSAGE FORMS:
- **Tablets (G):** 5 mg, 7.5 mg, 10 mg, 12.5 mg, 15 mg, 20 mg, 30 mg.
- **ER capsules (G):** 5 mg, 10 mg, 15 mg, 20 mg, 25 mg, 30 mg.
- **ER capsules (Mydayis):** 12.5 mg, 25 mg, 37.5 mg, 50 mg.

PEDIATRIC DOSAGE GUIDANCE:
- ADHD:
  - For both preparations: Initial dose should be 0.3 mg/kg/day, but shoot for a target dose of 1.0 mg/kg/day and maximum dose of 2 mg/kg/day.
  - IR (ages 3–5): Start 2.5 mg QAM, increase by 2.5 mg/day increments in weekly intervals, max 40 mg/day divided BID.
  - IR (ages 6–17): Start 5 mg QAM or BID, increase by 5 mg/day increments in weekly intervals, max 40 mg/day divided BID.
  - ER (ages 6–12): Start 5 mg QAM–10 mg QAM, increase by 5 mg/day–10 mg/day increments weekly, 30 mg/day.
  - ER (ages 13–17): Start 10 mg QAM, increase by 10 mg/day increments weekly, max 40 mg/day QAM in adolescents.
  - For Mydayis (adolescents 13–17 years), start 12.5 mg QAM, increase in increments of 12.5 mg/day weekly, to max 25 mg/day.
- Narcolepsy: Start 5 mg QAM (ages 6–11) or 10 mg QAM (ages 12–17), increase by 5 mg/day (ages 6–11) or 10 mg/day (ages 12–17) at weekly increments; max 60 mg/day.

MONITORING: Weight, height, BP/P; ECG.

COST: IR: $; ER: $$$

SIDE EFFECTS:
- Most common: insomnia, headache, decreased appetite, abdominal pain, weight loss, agitation.
- Serious but rare: See class warnings in chapter introduction.

MECHANISM, PHARMACOKINETICS, AND DRUG INTERACTIONS:
- Stimulant that inhibits reuptake of dopamine and norepinephrine.
- Metabolized primarily through CYP2D6; t ½: 9–14 hours. Duration of action: 6–8 hours (IR), 8–12 hours (XR).
- Avoid use with MAOIs, antacids. Caution with 2D6 inhibitors, which may increase stimulant effects.

EVIDENCE AND CLINICAL PEARLS:
- FDA-approved with many studies and long history of clinical use supporting its efficacy and safety, with a larger treatment effect size than non-stimulant medications.
- Each dose contains a mixture of amphetamine salts, resulting in a 75:25 ratio of dextro and levo isomers of amphetamine.
- When converting from IR to ER, use the same total daily dose, given QAM.
- Adderall may provide more of a "kick" than methylphenidate preparations. Roughly twice as potent (per mg) as methylphenidate.
- Mydayis is formulated with pH-dependent drug-releasing beads, with immediate release beads and delayed release beads that release drug at pH 5.5 and pH 7.0. Duration of effect may be up to 16 hours.
- Dextroamphetamine and mixed amphetamine salts are the only stimulants approved for children <6 years (approved for children >3 years), with the exception of Mydayis, which causes very high rates of side effects (insomnia, reduced appetite) in children <13 years and should only be used in children ≥13 years.

FUN FACT:
Was briefly pulled from the market in Canada in 2005 because of cardiac concerns.

BOTTOM LINE:
Adderall is effective but is probably the most abused and diverted of all stimulants, which is why we recommend starting most patients on methylphenidate instead.

Antidepressants

In contrast to the data available for adults, the evidence for efficacy and safety of antidepressants in children is less robust. Nonetheless, some studies, specifically the TADS (The Treatment for Adolescents With Depression Study) and TORDIA (Treatment of Resistant Depression in Adolescents), have shown that SSRIs can work for depression in adolescents, especially when combined with cognitive behavioral therapy.

In general, when faced with a child or adolescent with depression who has not responded to psychotherapy, we recommend starting with fluoxetine, because it has the most evidence for efficacy and safety. Other first-line options include sertraline and escitalopram. Paroxetine has fallen out of favor due to concerns about suicidality as a possible side effect and significant withdrawal symptoms.

If the first SSRI trial fails, rotate to a different SSRI. An SNRI trial (either venlafaxine or duloxetine) is reasonable after 2 failed SSRIs. SNRIs tend to have more side effects than SSRIs and potentially severe discontinuation symptoms.

Try bupropion for patients that have comorbid depression and ADHD, but remember that in patients with eating disorders, this drug causes a lowered seizure threshold. Mirtazapine and trazodone can be helpful for depressed and anxious patients with insomnia—but mirtazapine can cause substantial weight gain.

When antidepressants are not working well enough on their own, you can use augmenting agents, including atypical antipsychotics, lithium, and thyroid supplementation. However, there is very little research evidence supporting this practice in the pediatric population.

We rarely use tricyclics in kids, because of possible cardiac toxicity and other side effects. Nonetheless, consider them for particularly severe and unresponsive cases, or for patients with comorbid OCD, enuresis, insomnia, migraines, or poorly controlled headaches.

SIDE EFFECTS AND CLASS WARNINGS

- Black box warning of suicidality: All antidepressant medications come with a black box warning based off of a meta-analysis that demonstrated a 2-fold increase in suicidal thinking or behaviors in patients under 25 years of age. No completed suicides were demonstrated, and the suicidal parameters encompassed a broad range of definitions, including parasuicidal thoughts and behaviors. While the black box warning is a significant consideration, the pros of antidepressant treatment outweigh the cons in the majority of patients. Prior to the black box warning in 2004, the rate of suicide in the adolescent and young adult population was gradually decreasing while the number of SSRI prescriptions was rising. After the warning was placed, the number of SSRI prescriptions in this population dropped and the suicide rate increased. That being said, close monitoring and follow-up is imperative, particularly in the early stages of starting antidepressant medications, given the rare but significant risk of increased suicidality.

- SSRIs:
  - The most common side effects of SSRIs include GI symptoms of nausea and diarrhea, which are typically transient and resolve for the majority of patients after several days. These can be minimized by starting with lower doses than usual.
  - Sleep disruptions and intense dreams can occur.
  - Children and adolescents are more sensitive to activation and restlessness than adults.
  - Citalopram and (to a lesser extent) escitalopram increase QTc in a dose-dependent manner.
  - Increased bleeds due to platelet inhibition can occur with SSRIs and other serotonergic antidepressants.
  - Gradual tapers are required (with the exception of fluoxetine, given its long half-life) to avoid discontinuation symptoms, which most often occur with paroxetine. While not dangerous, discontinuation syndrome can be extremely uncomfortable and may include nausea, diarrhea, "brain zaps," headache, and irritability, to name a few symptoms.
- SNRIs:
  - Given their potential to increase blood pressure, closer blood pressure monitoring is required.
  - Gradual tapers are also required, in light of SNRIs' significant withdrawal symptoms.
- Other side effect considerations:
  - Serotonin syndrome can occur, particularly when using multiple serotonergic agents or serotonergic supplements such as St. John's wort or SAMe; if it occurs, it will require discontinuation of offending medications or supplements. Symptoms often present within a day of starting medication and can include sweating, GI symptoms, hyperthermia, tachycardia, increased blood pressure, confusion, and tremors, and can be life threatening; they will require immediate assessment and supportive care.
  - Risks of hypomania and mania need to be considered.
  - Sexual side effects can occur, including delayed orgasm/ejaculation and decreased sexual drive, which may be of concern to some adolescents—bupropion and mirtazapine are less likely to cause these problems.

TABLE 2: Antidepressants

Generic Name (Brand Name) Year FDA Approved [G] denotes generic availability	Relevant FDA Indication(s) (Pediatric indications in bold)	Available Strengths (mg)	Usual Dosage Range (starting–max) (mg) Pediatric unless specified
Selective serotonin reuptake inhibitor (SSRI)			
Citalopram [G] (Celexa) 1998	MDD	10, 20, 40, 10/5 mL	10–40
Escitalopram [G] (Lexapro) 2002	**MDD (12+ yrs)**, GAD	5, 10, 20, 5/5 mL	5–20
Fluoxetine [G] (Prozac) 1987	**MDD (8+ yrs), OCD (7+ yrs)**, panic disorder, bulimia, PMDD (as Sarafem)	10, 20, 40, 60, 20/5 mL 10, 20 (Sarafem)	10–60
Fluoxetine DR [G] (Prozac Weekly) 2001	MDD maintenance	90 DR	90 Qweek (adults)
Fluvoxamine [G] Luvox brand discontinued; generic only 1994	**OCD (8+ yrs)**	25, 50, 100	50–300
Fluvoxamine ER [G] (Luvox CR) 2008	OCD	100, 150 ER	100–300
Paroxetine [G] (Paxil) 1992 (Pexeva) 2003 (Brisdelle) 2013	MDD, OCD, panic disorder, social anxiety, GAD, PTSD, PMDD, menopausal hot flashes (as Brisdelle)	7.5 (Brisdelle), 10, 20, 30, 40, 10/5 mL	10–60
Paroxetine CR [G] (Paxil CR) 1999	MDD, panic disorder, social anxiety, PMDD	12.5, 25, 37.5 ER	12.5–62.5
Sertraline [G] (Zoloft) 1991	MDD, **OCD (6+ yrs)**, panic disorder, PTSD, PMDD, social anxiety	25, 50, 100, 20/mL	12.5–200
Serotonin norepinephrine reuptake inhibitor (SNRI)			
Desvenlafaxine [G] (Khedezla, Pristiq) 2008	MDD	25, 50, 100 ER	50–100 (adults)
Duloxetine [G] (Cymbalta) 2004	MDD, **GAD (7+ yrs)** (also diabetic peripheral neuropathy, fibromyalgia, chronic musculoskeletal pain)	20, 30, 40, 60 DR	30–120
Venlafaxine [G] 1993 Effexor brand discontinued; generic only	MDD	25, 37.5, 50, 75, 100	37.5–75
Venlafaxine ER [G] (Effexor XR) 1997	MDD, GAD, social anxiety disorder, panic disorder	37.5, 75, 150, 225 ER	37.5–225
Tricyclic antidepressant (TCA)			
Amitriptyline [G] Elavil brand discontinued; generic only 1961	MDD	10, 25, 50, 75, 100, 150	25–200
Clomipramine [G] (Anafranil) 1989	**OCD (10+ yrs)**	25, 50, 75	25–200
Desipramine [G] (Norpramin) 1964	MDD	10, 25, 50, 75, 100, 150	25–150

Generic Name (Brand Name) Year FDA Approved [G] denotes generic availability	Relevant FDA Indication(s) (Pediatric indications in bold)	Available Strengths (mg)	Usual Dosage Range (starting–max) (mg) Pediatric unless specified
Imipramine [G] Tofranil brand discontinued; generic only 1984	MDD	10, 25, 50, 75, 100, 125, 150	10–100
Nortriptyline [G] (Pamelor) 1977	MDD	10, 25, 50, 75, 10/5 mL	10–150
Monoamine oxidase inhibitor (MAOI)			
Selegiline transdermal (EMSAM) 2006	MDD	6, 9, 12/24h patch	6/24h–12/24h (adults)
Dopamine norepinephrine reuptake inhibitor			
Bupropion [G] (Wellbutrin) 1985	MDD	75, 100	100–450
Bupropion SR [G] (Wellbutrin SR) 1996	MDD, smoking cessation	100, 150, 200	100–400
Bupropion XL [G] (Wellbutrin XL, Forfivo XL) 2003	MDD, seasonal affective disorder	150, 300 (Wellbutrin XL), 450 (Forfivo XL)	150–450
Noradrenergic and specific serotonergic antidepressant (NaSSA)			
Mirtazapine [G] (Remeron) 1996	MDD	7.5, 15, 30, 45	7.5–45
Mirtazapine ODT [G] (Remeron SolTab) 2001	MDD	15, 30, 45	7.5–45
Serotonin reuptake inhibitor and 5-HT2A and 5-HT2C antagonist			
Trazodone [G] Desyrel brand discontinued; generic only 1981	MDD	50, 100, 150, 300	25–400

BUPROPION (Wellbutrin) Fact Sheet [G]

PEDIATRIC FDA INDICATIONS:
None.

ADULT FDA INDICATIONS:
Major depression; seasonal affective disorder; smoking cessation (as Zyban).

OFF-LABEL USES:
ADHD; sexual dysfunction; bipolar depression.

DOSAGE FORMS:
- **Tablets (G):** 75 mg, 100 mg.
- **SR tablets (G):** 100 mg, 150 mg, 200 mg.
- **ER tablets (G):** 150 mg, 300 mg; **Forfivo XL:** 450 mg.
- **ER tablets, hydrobromide salt formulation (Aplenzin):** 174 mg, 348 mg, 522 mg (equivalent to 150 mg, 300 mg, 450 mg, respectively).

PEDIATRIC DOSAGE GUIDANCE:
- Depression (target dose 300 mg/day):
  - IR: Start 37.5 mg or 75 mg BID, ↑ to TID after >3 days; max dose 450 mg/day, 150 mg/dose; separate doses by at least 6 hours to minimize seizure risk.
  - SR: Start 100 mg QAM, ↑ to 100 mg BID as early as fourth day; max dose 400 mg/day, 200 mg/dose; separate doses by at least 8 hours to minimize seizure risk.
  - ER: Start 150 mg QAM, ↑ to 300 mg QAM as early as fourth day; max dose 450 mg QAM.
- Smoking cessation: Start 100 mg SR QAM, titrate as needed.

MONITORING: No routine monitoring recommended unless clinical picture warrants.

COST: IR/SR/ER: $; Forfivo: $$$$; Aplenzin: $$$$$

SIDE EFFECTS:
- Most common: agitation, insomnia, headache, nausea, vomiting, tremor, tachycardia, dry mouth, weight loss.
- Serious but rare: seizures; risk higher with rapid and large dose increases and in patients at risk for seizures. Risk of seizure depends on dose and formulation: IR: 300 mg/day–450 mg/day (0.4%) vs 450 mg/day–600 mg/day (4%). SR/ER: 100 mg/day–300 mg/day (0.1%) vs 400 mg/day (0.4%). Do not chew, divide, or crush SR or ER tablets as risk of seizures may be increased.

MECHANISM, PHARMACOKINETICS, AND DRUG INTERACTIONS:
- Dopamine and norepinephrine receptor uptake inhibitor.
- Metabolized primarily through CYP2B6; inhibits CYP2D6; t ½: 21 hours.
- Avoid use with MAOIs.

EVIDENCE AND CLINICAL PEARLS:
- Although used clinically by some child psychiatrists, support for bupropion's efficacy in depression is based on 1 study in kids with comorbid ADHD and 1 open trial in adolescents with depression.
- For treatment of ADHD, a few head-to-head studies found bupropion to be equally effective as methylphenidate, but a large placebo-controlled trial found smaller effect sizes for bupropion.
- May be a particularly good option for kids with comorbid illness, such as ADHD or tobacco use disorder.
- There are only a few studies of bupropion for smoking cessation in adolescents. One study found bupropion provided no benefit when added to nicotine patches vs using patch alone. But another study showed improved quit rates (though lower than in adults) when combined with counseling vs counseling alone.
- Forfivo XL offers ease of use (1 pill a day) for patients taking 450 mg/day, but it is more expensive. Aplenzin brand could also be a 1-pill-a-day solution (522 mg is equivalent to 450 mg Wellbutrin) but otherwise doesn't offer any real advantage as a different salt (hydrobromide).
- Give ER dose as early in the morning as possible to minimize insomnia.
- Bupropion can cause false-positive urine test results for amphetamines.

NOT-SO-FUN FACT:
There have been case reports of teenagers, prisoners, and others snorting crushed tablets (believing the substance to be a stimulant), with subsequent seizures.

BOTTOM LINE:
Not a first-line antidepressant in kids, but may be useful for kids whose depression is associated with fatigue and poor concentration. Absence of sexual side effects and weight gain make this an appealing option for some. Although not effective for anxiety disorders, it is effective for the anxiety that often accompanies depression. The seizure risk is not a concern for most patients when dosed appropriately.

CITALOPRAM (Celexa) Fact Sheet [G]

PEDIATRIC FDA INDICATIONS:
None.

ADULT FDA INDICATIONS:
Major depression.

OFF-LABEL USES:
OCD; PTSD; social anxiety; GAD; panic disorder; PMDD.

DOSAGE FORMS:
- **Tablets (G):** 10 mg, 20 mg, 40 mg.
- **Oral solution (G):** 10 mg/5 mL.

PEDIATRIC DOSAGE GUIDANCE:
- Minimal dosing guidance in children and adolescents.
- Ages 7–11: Start 10 mg QD, increase by 5 mg/day increments every 1–2 weeks; max 40 mg/day.
- Ages 12–17: Start 10 mg or 20 mg QD, increase by 10 mg/day increments every 1–2 weeks; max 40 mg/day.

MONITORING: ECG in patients on >40 mg/day.

COST: $

SIDE EFFECTS:
- Most common: nausea, insomnia, anxiety, sexual side effects, apathy, headache.
- Serious but rare: hyponatremia, mainly in the elderly; gastrointestinal bleeding, especially when combined with NSAIDs such as ibuprofen.

MECHANISM, PHARMACOKINETICS, AND DRUG INTERACTIONS:
- Selective serotonin reuptake inhibitor.
- Metabolized primarily through CYP 2C19, 3A4; t ½: 35 hours.
- Avoid use with MAOIs (allow a 2-week washout period); avoid other serotonergic agents (serotonin syndrome).

EVIDENCE AND CLINICAL PEARLS:
- A 12-week randomized double-blind European study of 244 adolescents with depression found no significant difference in improvement between citalopram and placebo. When patients receiving psychotherapy were excluded from analysis, there were significantly higher response and remission rates with citalopram than placebo.
- Another 8-week randomized double-blind trial in 174 children and adolescents with depression found citalopram response rates low (36%), but significantly higher than placebo (24%).
- Citalopram's maximum daily dose was reduced to 40 mg/day by the FDA in August 2011 due to data suggesting increased QTc interval prolongation at doses >40 mg/day. Mean QTc interval prolongation at 60 mg/day was 18.5 msec (vs ziprasidone, which has been shown to increase this interval by 20.6 msec).
- Use lower doses and max 20 mg/day in patients deemed to be poor CYP 2C19 metabolizers.

FUN FACT:
A parody prescription drug commercial by the website *Funny or Die* is based on a combination of real-life clozapine and citalopram. The tagline is "DredLexa: the first depressant for rappers—sad music is better music."

BOTTOM LINE:
Citalopram does not have any pediatric indications, and its efficacy data are limited and modest; however, it is a reasonable second-line SSRI option.

DESVENLAFAXINE (Pristiq) Fact Sheet [G]

PEDIATRIC FDA INDICATIONS:
None.

ADULT FDA INDICATIONS:
Major depression.

OFF-LABEL USES:
Fibromyalgia; GAD; social anxiety disorder; panic disorder; PTSD; PMDD.

DOSAGE FORMS:
ER tablets (Pristiq, Khedezla, G): 25 mg, 50 mg, 100 mg.

PEDIATRIC DOSAGE GUIDANCE:
Start 25 mg QD. Increase to 50 mg QD based on response and tolerability. May increase to 100 mg QD in adolescents, but higher doses are generally not more effective and may be less well-tolerated.

MONITORING: Periodic BP.

COST: $$; Khedezla: $$$

SIDE EFFECTS:
- Most common: nausea, dizziness, insomnia, excessive sweating, constipation, dry mouth, somnolence, decreased appetite, anxiety, and sexual side effects.
- Serious but rare: dose-related increases in systolic and diastolic blood pressure (as likely with Pristiq as Effexor). Monitor BP regularly, and if increases are sustained, consider reducing dose or discontinuing.

MECHANISM, PHARMACOKINETICS, AND DRUG INTERACTIONS:
- Serotonin and norepinephrine reuptake inhibitor.
- Active metabolite of venlafaxine, metabolized primarily through conjugation and oxidation via CYP3A4 (minor). Minimally inhibits CYP2D6; t ½: 11 hours.
- Avoid use with MAOIs and other serotonergic medications. Not likely to cause other clinically significant interactions.

EVIDENCE AND CLINICAL PEARLS:
- Minimal data in kids with depression (1 open-label study of 20 children and 20 adolescents that looked at safety and tolerability only, not efficacy).
- A recent randomized double-blind placebo-controlled study of over 300 kids with depression showed desvenlafaxine was no better than placebo.
- Desvenlafaxine has not been shown to be any more effective than venlafaxine. Unlike venlafaxine, increasing the dose of desvenlafaxine beyond the recommended 50 mg/day likely does not improve response, but does increase side effects.
- Claims of fewer drug interactions with desvenlafaxine are likely unimportant for the majority of patients as the risk of clinically significant interactions with venlafaxine is already quite low.
- Desvenlafaxine is available in 2 forms: a succinate salt (Pristiq) and a base (Khedezla). Aside from small differences in half-life, there is no difference between these products—all efficacy studies were based on the original Pristiq studies.

FUN FACT:
Desvenlafaxine's manufacturer withdrew its application for approval in the European Union, where regulatory bodies had said that desvenlafaxine was likely less effective than venlafaxine with no advantages in terms of safety and tolerability.

BOTTOM LINE:
There are no clear advantages to using desvenlafaxine over other agents, particularly venlafaxine XR. Given minimal data in kids, we'd stick with venlafaxine if we want to go with an SNRI.

DULOXETINE (Cymbalta) Fact Sheet [G]

PEDIATRIC FDA INDICATIONS:
Generalized anxiety disorder (7–17 years).

ADULT FDA INDICATIONS:
Major depression; generalized anxiety disorder; diabetic peripheral neuropathic pain; fibromyalgia; chronic musculoskeletal pain (including osteoarthritis and chronic low back pain).

OFF-LABEL USES:
Other neuropathic or chronic pain disorders; other anxiety disorders; stress urinary incontinence.

DOSAGE FORMS:
Capsules (delayed release) (G): 20 mg, 30 mg, 40 mg, 60 mg.

PEDIATRIC DOSAGE GUIDANCE:
- GAD: Start 30 mg QD, increase by 30 mg/day after 2 weeks; max dose 60 mg QD.
- Depression: Minimal data in kids; follow GAD dosing recommendations.

MONITORING: Periodic BP.

COST: $

SIDE EFFECTS:
- Most common: nausea, dry mouth, constipation, diarrhea, decreased appetite, vomiting, fatigue, insomnia, dizziness, agitation, sweating, headache, urinary hesitation, and sexual side effects.
- Serious but rare: Rare cases of hepatic failure (including fatalities) have been reported (too rare to require routine LFTs in all patients). Hepatitis with abdominal pain, hepatomegaly, elevated transaminases >20 times normal, with and without jaundice observed. May cause orthostatic hypotension or syncope, especially in first week of therapy and after dose increases. Urinary retention reported; hospitalization and/or catheterization were necessary in some cases.

MECHANISM, PHARMACOKINETICS, AND DRUG INTERACTIONS:
- Serotonin and norepinephrine reuptake inhibitor.
- Metabolized primarily through CYP1A2 and 2D6; inhibitor of CYP2D6; t ½: 12 hours.
- Avoid use with MAOIs and other serotonergic medications. Caution with drugs metabolized by CYP2D6 (eg, paroxetine, fluoxetine, aripiprazole, iloperidone, risperidone, atomoxetine, beta blockers) as their levels may be increased. Potent inhibitors of CYP2D6 (eg, paroxetine, fluoxetine, quinidine) and CYP1A2 (eg, fluvoxamine, ciprofloxacin) may increase duloxetine levels.

EVIDENCE AND CLINICAL PEARLS:
- Two placebo-controlled studies of 8000 kids with depression didn't show efficacy. Two safety studies showed expected side effects in kids of increased BP and pulse, nausea, and headache.
- Since capsules are delayed release, they should be swallowed whole; do not chew or crush. Although the manufacturer does not recommend opening the capsules, their contents may be sprinkled on applesauce or in apple juice and swallowed immediately.
- Avoid in patients with a history of heavy alcohol use or chronic hepatic disease because of the possibility that duloxetine and alcohol may interact, causing hepatic injury, or the possibility that duloxetine may aggravate preexisting hepatic disease.

FUN FACT:
Duloxetine is approved in Europe for stress urinary incontinence, but the FDA refused this indication in the US because of concerns regarding liver toxicity and potential suicidal ideation.

BOTTOM LINE:
Minimal (and negative) data and possibly more side effects versus SSRIs (BP, P) relegate this to second- or third-line status for treating kids with depression. But consider in kids with GAD or in those with depression who have failed alternatives or who also have comorbid pain disorders.

ESCITALOPRAM (Lexapro) Fact Sheet [G]

PEDIATRIC FDA INDICATIONS:
Major depression (12+ years).

ADULT FDA INDICATIONS:
Major depression; GAD.

OFF-LABEL USES:
OCD; PTSD; social anxiety; panic disorder; PMDD; autism.

DOSAGE FORMS:
- **Tablets (G):** 5 mg, 10 mg, 20 mg.
- **Oral solution (G):** 5 mg/5 mL.

PEDIATRIC DOSAGE GUIDANCE:
- Ages 6–9: Start 2.5 mg QD, increase by 5 mg/day increments weekly; max 20 mg/day.
- Ages 10–17: Start 5 mg QD, increase by 5–10 mg/day increments weekly; max 20 mg/day.

MONITORING: ECG in patients on >20 mg/day.

COST: $; liquid: $$

SIDE EFFECTS:
- Most common: nausea, insomnia, anxiety, sedation, sexual side effects, weight gain, apathy, headache.
- Serious but rare: hyponatremia, mainly in the elderly; gastrointestinal bleeding, especially when combined with NSAIDs such as ibuprofen.

MECHANISM, PHARMACOKINETICS, AND DRUG INTERACTIONS:
- Selective serotonin reuptake inhibitor.
- Metabolized primarily through CYP 2C19, 3A4; t ½: 27–32 hours.
- Avoid use with MAOIs (allow a 2-week washout period); avoid other serotonergic agents (serotonin syndrome).

EVIDENCE AND CLINICAL PEARLS:
- An 8-week randomized clinical trial of 268 children (ages 6–17) with depression failed to find a significant difference between escitalopram and placebo on primary outcome measures. When data analysis included only adolescent subjects, there was a significant difference in favor of escitalopram.
- Another 8-week randomized clinical trial of 312 adolescents showed only a small to medium effect size (0.27) on primary outcome measures of depression.
- FDA approval for adolescents with depression aged 12 and over is based on 1 randomized double-blind placebo-controlled study in pediatric depression showing significantly greater efficacy compared to placebo.
- Escitalopram (which is purified from the racemic mixture, citalopram) is considered the "purest" SSRI and has few, if any, drug-drug interactions.

FUN FACT:
In his rap song "FML," Kanye West refers to "nothing crazier" than when "he off his Lexapro."

BOTTOM LINE:
Although only 1 of 3 randomized controlled trials led to FDA approval in adolescents, you may consider escitalopram a first-line agent, particularly in adolescents with depression and anxiety disorders. Efficacy of escitalopram in OCD and other anxiety disorders has not been established; stick to fluoxetine and sertraline.

FLUOXETINE (Prozac) Fact Sheet [G]

PEDIATRIC FDA INDICATIONS:
Major depression (8+ years), **OCD** (7+ years).

ADULT FDA INDICATIONS:
Major depression; OCD; panic disorder; bulimia; PMDD (as Sarafem).

OFF-LABEL USES:
PTSD; social anxiety; cataplexy.

DOSAGE FORMS:
- **Capsules (G):** 10 mg, 20 mg, 40 mg.
- **Tablets (Sarafem, G):** 10 mg, 20 mg, 60 mg.
- **DR capsules (Prozac Weekly, G):** 90 mg.
- **Oral solution (G):** 20 mg/5 mL.

PEDIATRIC DOSAGE GUIDANCE:
- Age 6–7: Start 5 mg QD, increase by 5 mg/day increments weekly; max 30 mg/day.
- Age 8–17: Start 10 mg QD, increase by 10 mg/day increments weekly; max 60 mg/day.
- Many children and adolescents will show good treatment response at 10 mg/day.

MONITORING: No routine monitoring recommended unless clinical picture warrants.

COST: $; DR capsule: $$$

SIDE EFFECTS:
- Most common: nausea, insomnia, anxiety, sexual side effects, apathy, headache.
- Serious but rare: hyponatremia, mainly in the elderly; gastrointestinal bleeding, especially when combined with NSAIDs such as ibuprofen.

MECHANISM, PHARMACOKINETICS, AND DRUG INTERACTIONS:
- Selective serotonin reuptake inhibitor.
- Metabolized primarily through CYP 2D6; t ½: 4–6 days (9 days for norfluoxetine metabolite). Potent CYP 2C9/19, 2D6 inhibitor; moderate CYP 3A4 inhibitor.
- Avoid use with MAOIs (allow a 5-week washout period); avoid other serotonergic agents (serotonin syndrome).

EVIDENCE AND CLINICAL PEARLS:
- Most studied SSRI in kids and the only antidepressant approved for treating depression in younger children.
- Two large randomized double-blind placebo-controlled trials showing significantly greater efficacy for depression compared to placebo led to FDA indication in kids 8 and older.
- Fluoxetine is favored in patients who could use some activation; it is most likely to cause insomnia, anxiety, and decreased appetite.
- Generally, higher doses of SSRIs are required for treating OCD.

FUN FACT:
According to *National Geographic*, shrimp exposed to traces of fluoxetine swim in brighter areas, making them more vulnerable to predators. This fact is not so fun for the shrimp.

BOTTOM LINE:
Consider fluoxetine a first-line agent for kids with depression and anxiety disorders.

FLUVOXAMINE (Luvox) Fact Sheet [G]

PEDIATRIC FDA INDICATIONS:
OCD (8+ years).

ADULT FDA INDICATIONS:
OCD.

OFF-LABEL USES:
Major depression; panic disorder; GAD; PTSD.

DOSAGE FORMS:
- **Tablets (G):** 25 mg, 50 mg, 100 mg.
- **ER capsules (G):** 100 mg, 150 mg.

PEDIATRIC DOSAGE GUIDANCE:
Start 25 mg QHS, increase by 25 mg/day increments weekly; max 200 mg/day in ages 8–11 and 300 mg/day in ages >11. Doses >50 mg/day should be divided BID.

MONITORING: No routine monitoring recommended unless clinical picture warrants.

COST: $; ER: $$$

SIDE EFFECTS:
- Most common: nausea, sedation, sexual side effects, weight gain, apathy, headache.
- Serious but rare: hyponatremia, mainly in the elderly; gastrointestinal bleeding, especially when combined with NSAIDs such as ibuprofen.

MECHANISM, PHARMACOKINETICS, AND DRUG INTERACTIONS:
- Selective serotonin reuptake inhibitor.
- Metabolized primarily through CYP 1A2, 2D6; t ½: 16 hours. Potent CYP 1A2, 2C9/19, 3A4 inhibitor.
- Avoid use with MAOIs (allow a 2-week washout period); avoid other serotonergic agents (serotonin syndrome).

EVIDENCE AND CLINICAL PEARLS:
- An 8-week placebo-controlled trial of 128 children (6–17 years) with social phobia, separation anxiety disorder, or generalized anxiety disorder found significantly greater improvement on anxiety measure with fluvoxamine compared to placebo.
- A 10-week placebo-controlled trial of 120 children and adolescents (8–17 years) with OCD showed significantly higher reduction in Children's Yale-Brown Obsessive Compulsive Scale scores with fluvoxamine compared to placebo.
- There are no high-quality studies of fluvoxamine in children with depression.
- Fluvoxamine is used less often due to twice-daily dosing, risk for drug interactions, and fewer data for uses other than OCD, even though it's likely just as effective as other SSRIs.
- Discontinuation symptoms tend to be worse with fluvoxamine compared to other SSRIs.
- Generally, higher doses of SSRIs are required for treating OCD.

FUN FACT:
Families of victims of the Columbine shooting sued Luvox's manufacturer after it was revealed one of the shooters was taking this antidepressant.

BOTTOM LINE:
Fluvoxamine was the first SSRI approved for OCD in children as young as 8. We favor fluoxetine and sertraline for ease of dosing, better tolerability, generally lower drug interaction potential, and lower likelihood for discontinuation syndrome.

MIRTAZAPINE (Remeron) Fact Sheet [G]

PEDIATRIC FDA INDICATIONS:
None.

ADULT FDA INDICATIONS:
Major depression.

OFF-LABEL USES:
Panic disorder; PTSD; generalized anxiety disorder; insomnia; nausea; appetite stimulant.

DOSAGE FORMS:
- **Tablets (G):** 7.5 mg, 15 mg, 30 mg, 45 mg.
- **Orally disintegrating tablets (G):** 15 mg, 30 mg, 45 mg.

PEDIATRIC DOSAGE GUIDANCE:
- Very limited dosing guidance in children and adolescents.
- Start 7.5 mg or 15 mg QHS, ↑ by 15 mg/day every 1–2 weeks. Max 45 mg/day.

MONITORING: Weight.

COST: $; ODT: $

SIDE EFFECTS:
- Most common: somnolence, increased appetite, weight gain, perhaps offset by stimulating effects of higher dosages.
- Serious but rare: agranulocytosis or severe neutropenia (with or without infection) reported very rarely.

MECHANISM, PHARMACOKINETICS, AND DRUG INTERACTIONS:
- Noradrenergic (via central presynaptic alpha-2 adrenergic receptor antagonist activity) and specific serotonergic (via postsynaptic 5HT2 and 5HT3 antagonist effects) antidepressant.
- Metabolized primarily through CYP1A2, 2D6, and 3A4; t ½: 20–40 hours.
- Avoid use with MAOIs and other serotonergic agents. Caution with inducers of 1A2 or 3A4 (eg, carbamazepine), which could reduce efficacy of mirtazapine.

EVIDENCE AND CLINICAL PEARLS:
- Two unpublished 8-week randomized trials of mirtazapine 15–45 mg/day in outpatient children and adolescents with depression found no significant reduction in depressive symptoms compared to placebo.
- One open-label 85-day study of mirtazapine 30–45 mg/day in 24 adolescents with depression showed marked efficacy on depression, anxiety, and sleep as well as good tolerability (sedation, weight gain, and increased appetite were most common).
- Twenty-six subjects with pervasive developmental disorder (PDD) between age 4–24 years were treated with mirtazapine 7.5 mg–45 mg/day in an open-label trial, showing only modest benefit for symptoms associated with autism and other PDD.
- If patients experience too much sedation at initial lower dose, increase dose; mirtazapine has increased noradrenergic effect relative to antihistaminergic effect at higher doses.

FUN FACT:
Esmirtazapine, the (S)-enantiomer, was under development for the treatment of insomnia and hot flashes associated with menopause, but the company pulled the plug in 2010.

BOTTOM LINE:
Second- or third-line agent due to lack of data. Weight gain and sedation may limit its use in many kids. It may be useful in depressed patients with anxiety or insomnia, those who have had sexual side effects with other antidepressants, and those who may benefit from appetite stimulation.

PAROXETINE (Paxil, Pexeva) Fact Sheet [G]

PEDIATRIC FDA INDICATIONS:
None.

ADULT FDA INDICATIONS:
Major depression; OCD; panic disorder; social anxiety; GAD; PTSD; PMDD; menopausal hot flashes (as Brisdelle).

OFF-LABEL USES:
Premature ejaculation.

DOSAGE FORMS:
- **Tablets (G):** 10 mg, 20 mg, 30 mg, 40 mg.
- **Oral solution:** 10 mg/5 mL.
- **ER tablets (G):** 12.5 mg, 25 mg, 37.5 mg.
- **Capsules (Brisdelle, G):** 7.5 mg.

PEDIATRIC DOSAGE GUIDANCE:
- Minimal dosing guidance in children and adolescents.
- Start 10 mg QD, increase by 10 mg/day increments every 1–2 weeks; max 60 mg/day.
- Start CR 12.5 mg QD, increase by 12.5 mg/day increments every 1–2 weeks; max 62.5 mg/day.

MONITORING: No routine monitoring recommended unless clinical picture warrants.

COST: $; liquid: $$$$; CR: $$

SIDE EFFECTS:
- Most common: nausea, sedation, anxiety, constipation, sexual side effects, weight gain, apathy, headache.
- Serious but rare: hyponatremia, mainly in the elderly; gastrointestinal bleeding, especially when combined with NSAIDs such as ibuprofen.

MECHANISM, PHARMACOKINETICS, AND DRUG INTERACTIONS:
- Selective serotonin reuptake inhibitor.
- Metabolized primarily through CYP 2D6; t ½: 21 hours. Potent CYP 2D6 inhibitor.
- Avoid use with MAOIs (allow a 2-week washout period); avoid other serotonergic agents (serotonin syndrome).

EVIDENCE AND CLINICAL PEARLS:
- Study 329, a 2001 study comparing paroxetine to imipramine in kids with depression, became controversial when it was found not only that the study had been ghostwritten by a PR firm hired by the drug manufacturer, but also that it made inappropriate claims about efficacy and downplayed safety concerns. A re-analysis published in 2015 found that neither paroxetine nor imipramine were better than placebo for depression and that paroxetine patients experienced more suicidal ideation and behavior while imipramine patients experienced more cardiovascular problems.
- A meta-analysis of 4 paroxetine trials in kids with depression found similar response and remission rates with placebo.
- Of the SSRIs, paroxetine is least favored due to its side effect profile (greatest sexual side effects, weight gain, sedation, constipation) and drug interaction profile.
- Discontinuation symptoms tend to be worse with paroxetine compared to other SSRIs.

FUN FACT:
New Scientist wrote in 2015: "You may never have heard of it, but Study 329 changed medicine."

BOTTOM LINE:
Lack of efficacy, side effects, and discontinuation symptoms make paroxetine less appealing for children with depression.

SELEGILINE TRANSDERMAL (EMSAM) Fact Sheet

PEDIATRIC FDA INDICATIONS:
None.

ADULT FDA INDICATIONS:
Major depression.

OFF-LABEL USES:
Treatment-resistant depression; panic disorder; treatment-resistant anxiety disorders.

DOSAGE FORMS:
Transdermal patch: 6 mg, 9 mg, 12 mg/24 hour patch.

PEDIATRIC DOSAGE GUIDANCE:
- No dosing guidance in children and adolescents.
- Start 6 mg/24 hours QD; may ↑ in increments of 3 mg/24 hours every 4 weeks, up to max 12 mg/24 hours.
- Apply to clean, dry, intact skin on upper torso (below neck and above waist), upper thigh, or outer surface of upper arm; apply at the same time each day and rotate application sites; wash hands with soap and water after handling; avoid touching sticky side of patch.

MONITORING: No routine monitoring recommended unless clinical picture warrants.

COST: $$$$

SIDE EFFECTS:
- Most common: headache, insomnia, application site reaction, hypotension, diarrhea, dry mouth.
- Serious but rare: orthostatic hypotension; caution in patients at risk (elderly, cerebrovascular disease, cardiovascular disease, hypovolemia).

MECHANISM, PHARMACOKINETICS, AND DRUG INTERACTIONS:
- Non-selective monoamine oxidase inhibitor.
- Metabolized primarily through CYP2B6 (also 2C9, 3A4/5) to active (N-desmethylselegiline, amphetamine, methamphetamine) and inactive metabolites; t ½: 18–25 hours.
- Avoid with other antidepressants, serotonergic agents, stimulants, sympathomimetics, dextromethorphan, disulfiram, meperidine, and carbamazepine. Do not use within 5 weeks of fluoxetine discontinuation or 2 weeks of other antidepressant discontinuation. Discontinue at least 10 days prior to elective surgery. Antihypertensives may exaggerate hypotensive effects. For doses higher than 6 mg, avoid use with foods or supplements high in tyramine, tryptophan, phenylalanine, or tyrosine.
- Wait 2 weeks after discontinuing transdermal selegiline before initiating therapy with serotonergic or any other contraindicated drug.

EVIDENCE AND CLINICAL PEARLS:
- Only 1 study in adolescents with depression, which showed that it was well-tolerated but had no benefit over placebo.
- Oral selegiline (Eldepryl) used in Parkinson's disease (≤10 mg/day) is a selective inhibitor of MAO-B, which metabolizes dopamine. When used transdermally as EMSAM, selegiline achieves higher blood levels and non-selectively inhibits both MAO-A and MAO-B. Its antidepressant effect is thought to be due to its MAO-A inhibition, which blocks the breakdown of other centrally active neurotransmitters (norepinephrine, serotonin).
- When using 6 mg/day patch, no special diet required. When using higher doses, a tyramine-restricted diet should be followed.
- Patch may contain conducting metal (eg, aluminum); avoid exposure of application site to external heat source, which may increase the amount of drug absorbed.

FUN FACT:
Named "EMSAM" after Emily and Samuel, the children of the CEO of Somerset Pharmaceuticals (original manufacturer).

BOTTOM LINE:
Minimal efficacy data in pediatric patients, and likelihood that adolescents in particular may not follow diet restrictions, relegate this to third-line status.

SERTRALINE (Zoloft) Fact Sheet [G]

PEDIATRIC FDA INDICATIONS:
OCD (6+ years).

ADULT FDA INDICATIONS:
Major depression; panic disorder; PTSD; PMDD; social anxiety.

OFF-LABEL USES:
Generalized anxiety disorder.

DOSAGE FORMS:
- **Tablets (G):** 25 mg, 50 mg, 100 mg.
- **Oral solution (G):** 20 mg/mL.

PEDIATRIC DOSAGE GUIDANCE:
- Age 6–12: Start 12.5 mg–25 mg QD, increase by 25–50 mg/day increments weekly; max 200 mg/day.
- Age 13–17: Start 25 mg–50 mg QD, increase by 25–50 mg/day increments weekly; max 200 mg/day.

MONITORING: No routine monitoring recommended unless clinical picture warrants.

COST: $

SIDE EFFECTS:
- Most common: nausea, insomnia, anxiety, apathy, headache.
- Serious but rare: hyponatremia, mainly in the elderly; gastrointestinal bleeding, especially when combined with NSAIDs such as ibuprofen.

MECHANISM, PHARMACOKINETICS, AND DRUG INTERACTIONS:
- Selective serotonin reuptake inhibitor.
- Metabolized primarily through CYP 2C19 (also 2D6, 3A4); t ½: 26 hours. At higher doses, may moderately inhibit CYP 2D6.
- Avoid use with MAOIs (allow a 2-week washout period); avoid other serotonergic agents (serotonin syndrome).

EVIDENCE AND CLINICAL PEARLS:
- FDA approval for OCD in children is based on 2 positive trials. One was a 12-week randomized study of 112 kids ages 7–17 with OCD that found both CBT alone and sertraline alone to be significantly more effective than placebo, and the combination to be significantly more effective than either alone. The second was a 12-week randomized controlled trial of 187 kids (ages 6–18) that found sertraline was significantly more effective than placebo on all OCD outcome measures.
- Sertraline is also significantly more effective than placebo in children with depression based on a pooled analysis of two 10-week randomized studies of 364 patients (69% of sertraline vs 59% of placebo kids had >40% reduction of baseline symptoms).
- Generally, higher doses of SSRIs are required for treating OCD.

FUN FACT:
Zoloft is often remembered for the TV ad with the narration "You know when the world seems like a sad and lonely place?" An animated blob goes from shaky and isolated to happy; led by an orange butterfly, it bounces, smiles, and emerges from a cave to join 2 other blobs.

BOTTOM LINE:
Consider sertraline a first-line agent for kids with depression and anxiety disorders.

TRAZODONE Fact Sheet [G]

PEDIATRIC FDA INDICATIONS:
None.

ADULT FDA INDICATIONS:
Major depression.

OFF-LABEL USES:
Insomnia; anxiety.

DOSAGE FORMS:
Tablets (G): 50 mg, 100 mg, 150 mg, 300 mg (scored).

PEDIATRIC DOSAGE GUIDANCE:
- Depression:
  - Ages 6–12: Start 1.5 mg/kg/day–2 mg/kg/day divided TID; ↑ every 3–4 days to response; max 6 mg/kg/day.
  - Ages 13–17: Start 25 mg BID–TID, increase dose every 3–4 days; max dose 6 mg/kg/day up to 400 mg/day.
- Insomnia (off-label): Start 25 mg QHS; may ↑ by 25 mg increments every 2 weeks, up to 200 mg QHS.

MONITORING: No routine monitoring recommended unless clinical picture warrants.

COST: $

SIDE EFFECTS:
- Most common: drowsiness, dry mouth, dizziness or lightheadedness, orthostatic hypotension, headache, blurred vision, nausea, or vomiting.
- Serious but rare: reports of priapism (painful erection >6 hours in duration); may require surgical or pharmacologic (eg, epinephrine) intervention and may result in impotence or permanent impairment of erectile function. Orthostatic hypotension and syncope reported (less at hypnotic doses).

MECHANISM, PHARMACOKINETICS, AND DRUG INTERACTIONS:
- Serotonin reuptake inhibitor, alpha-1 adrenergic receptor antagonist, and serotonin 5HT2A and 5HT2C receptor antagonist.
- Metabolized primarily through CYP3A4 to active metabolite (mCPP), which in turn is metabolized by 2D6; induces P-glycoprotein; t ½: 7–10 hours.
- Avoid use with MAOIs.

EVIDENCE AND CLINICAL PEARLS:
- Although efficacy data in kids are lacking, fairly commonly used to manage sleep in kids.
- If daytime drowsiness occurs, administer the majority of dosage at bedtime or ↓ dose.
- Trazodone's hypnotic effects are not due to anticholinergic or antihistaminergic effects.
- IR formulation rarely used as antidepressant due to risk for over-sedation and orthostasis at therapeutic doses; majority of IR use currently is for insomnia.

FUN FACT:
As a consequence of the production of mCPP as a metabolite, patients taking trazodone may test positive on urine tests for the presence of MDMA (ecstasy).

BOTTOM LINE:
Limited evidence to support its use, but fairly commonly used for insomnia in clinical practice.

TRICYCLIC ANTIDEPRESSANTS (TCAs) Fact Sheet [G]

PEDIATRIC FDA INDICATIONS:
Obsessive compulsive disorder (clomipramine, 10–17 years); **nocturnal enuresis** (imipramine, 6–17 years).

ADULT FDA INDICATIONS:
Major depression; obsessive compulsive disorder (OCD).

OFF-LABEL USES:
Headache; neuropathic pain; fibromyalgia; anxiety disorders; insomnia; cataplexy; sleep terrors; sleepwalking.

DOSAGE FORMS:
- **Amitriptyline tablets (G):** 10 mg, 25 mg, 50 mg, 75 mg, 100 mg, 150 mg.
- **Clomipramine capsules (Anafranil, G):** 25 mg, 50 mg, 75 mg.
- **Desipramine tablets (Norpramin, G):** 10 mg, 25 mg, 50 mg, 75 mg, 100 mg, 150 mg.
- **Imipramine tablets and capsules (G):** 10 mg, 25 mg, 50 mg, 75 mg, 100 mg, 125 mg, 150 mg.
- **Nortriptyline capsules (Pamelor, G):** 10 mg, 25 mg, 50 mg, 75 mg, and 10 mg/5 mL oral solution.

PEDIATRIC DOSAGE GUIDANCE:
- Amitriptyline or imipramine: For ages 6–12, start 1 mg/kg/day divided TID, increase by 0.5 mg/kg/day every 3 days; max 5 mg/kg/day or 200 mg/day. For ages 3–17, start 25 mg–50 mg QHS or divided TID, ↑ by 10 mg/day–25 mg/day intervals every 3 days to max 200 mg/day.
- Clomipramine: Start 25 mg QHS and ↑ by 25 mg/day every 4–7 days to max 200 mg/day.
- Desipramine: Start 25 mg QHS, ↑ by 25 mg/day intervals every 4–7 days to max 150 mg/day.
- Nortriptyline: For ages 6–12, start 1 mg/kg/day divided TID, increase by 0.5 mg/kg/day every 3 days; max 150 mg/day. For ages 13–17, start 25 mg–50 mg QHS or divided TID, ↑ by 10 mg/day–50 mg/day intervals every 3 days to max 150 mg/day.
- For enuresis: imipramine 10 mg QHS, increase by 10 mg/day increments every 1–2 weeks; max 75 mg/day.

MONITORING: ECG in patients at risk.

COST: clomipramine: $$$; all others: $

SIDE EFFECTS:
- Most common: sedation, dry mouth, constipation, weight gain, sexual side effects, urinary hesitation, blurred vision.
- Serious but rare: seizure; cardiac effects including orthostasis, arrhythmias, QT prolongation, AV block.

MECHANISM, PHARMACOKINETICS, AND DRUG INTERACTIONS:
- Serotonin and norepinephrine reuptake inhibitor.
- Metabolized primarily through liver, likely CYP2D6 primarily; t ½: 18–44 hours.
- Avoid use with other serotonergic antidepressants or agents with hypotensive or anticholinergic effects.

EVIDENCE AND CLINICAL PEARLS:
- Only 1 small study (n = 30), of nearly a dozen placebo-controlled studies of TCAs in children and adolescents, showed positive results. A meta-analysis similarly found no efficacy for depression in kids.
- Nortriptyline improved symptoms of ADHD in kids, but the effect was not as robust as with stimulants.
- Clomipramine can be very effective in childhood OCD but has a greater side effect burden.
- TCAs reduce frequency of bedwetting in kids with enuresis, but benefits are not sustained after medication is discontinued. Behavioral interventions and alarms are preferred.
- Divided doses (BID to TID) may help with tolerability initially; convert to QHS to minimize daytime sedation.
- Overdose toxicity with potentially serious cardiac effects or fatality with as little as 10-day supply. Sudden death reported in several patients taking therapeutic doses of TCAs. Avoid use in those at risk.

FUN FACT:
Imipramine was the first antidepressant approved in the US, developed by tweaking the molecular structure of the antipsychotic Thorazine. It didn't work for psychosis, but was the first wonder drug for depression and anxiety.

BOTTOM LINE:
Not commonly used due to side effects and toxicity risk; however, TCAs should be considered for kids who do not respond to other antidepressants.

VENLAFAXINE (Effexor XR) Fact Sheet [G]

PEDIATRIC FDA INDICATIONS:
None.

ADULT FDA INDICATIONS:
Major depression; social anxiety disorder; GAD; panic disorder.

OFF-LABEL USES:
PTSD; PMDD; vasomotor symptoms of menopause; diabetic peripheral neuropathy; fibromyalgia.

DOSAGE FORMS:
- **Tablets (G):** 25 mg, 37.5 mg, 50 mg, 75 mg, 100 mg (scored).
- **ER tablets (G):** 37.5 mg, 75 mg, 150 mg, 225 mg.

PEDIATRIC DOSAGE GUIDANCE:
- Depression:
  - Ages 8–12: Start 12.5 mg QD or 37.5 mg as XR once daily; ↑ dose by 12.5 mg/day (IR) or 37.5 mg/day (XR) increments at intervals of 4 or more days; max 75 mg/day (divided TID for IR). IR may be switched to nearest equivalent daily dose of XR QD.
  - Ages 13–17: Start 25 mg QD or 37.5 mg as XR QD, ↑ dose by 25 mg/day (IR) or 37.5 mg/day (XR) increments at intervals of 4 or more days; max 75 mg/day (divided TID for IR). ER max dose 225 mg/day in adolescents.
- Anxiety:
  - XR: Start 37.5 mg QD, ↑ by 37.5 mg/day at weekly intervals; max 225 mg/day.

MONITORING: Periodic BP.

COST: IR: $; ER: $

SIDE EFFECTS:
- Most common: anorexia, constipation, dizziness, dry mouth, nausea, nervousness, somnolence, sweating, sexual side effects, headache, insomnia.
- Serious but rare: sustained, dose-related hypertension reported. May cause hyponatremia or SIADH; use with caution in patients who are volume-depleted, elderly, or taking diuretics.

MECHANISM, PHARMACOKINETICS, AND DRUG INTERACTIONS:
- Serotonin and norepinephrine reuptake inhibitor.
- Metabolized primarily through CYP2D6 to O-desmethylvenlafaxine (ODV), major active metabolite (an SNRI, marketed as Pristiq), and also by CYP3A4; t ½: 5 hours (11 hours for ODV).
- Avoid use with MAOIs and other serotonergic agents. Caution with CYP2D6 or 3A4 inhibitors, which may increase venlafaxine levels. Inhibits CYP2D6.

EVIDENCE AND CLINICAL PEARLS
- An open study suggested venlafaxine may be effective for adolescent depression, but 2 randomized controlled studies in kids (7–17 years) with depression found venlafaxine was no better than placebo.
- Two randomized double-blind placebo-controlled studies in more than 300 children and adolescents with GAD showed greater improvement with venlafaxine compared to placebo. Efficacy has been shown in social phobia as well.
- For patients with nausea, start at lower dose, titrate more slowly, and give with food.
- May cause false positive for PCP in a urine drug screen.
- Increase in blood pressure much more likely in doses >225 mg/day.
- Significant discontinuation syndrome, even with XR formulation. Taper by no more than 75 mg/week to discontinue.

FUN FACT:
Venlafaxine is structurally related to the atypical opioid analgesic tramadol (Ultram), itself a serotonergic agent, but not to any other antidepressant drugs.

BOTTOM LINE:
Fewer data than SSRIs places venlafaxine in the second-line category for both depression and GAD in kids.

Antipsychotics

Antipsychotics are potent medications that have been likened to chemotherapy for the brain. Their use in children and adolescents can yield impressive results, but they can also lead to very problematic side effects. It is important to stay current on research trends and take clinical situations one at a time. Try not to be swayed by occasional cases of spectacular improvement or extreme side effects. Document your rationale, including possible risks and benefits. Most importantly, advocate for comprehensive care, which can reduce the need for these medications and their attendant risks.

Here are some tips on using antipsychotics in children and adolescents.

EFFICACY

Antipsychotics have many uses, both on and off label. They are FDA-approved (marked by an *) or have some evidence supporting use for the following indications in children and adolescents:

- Positive and negative psychotic symptoms*
- Irritability in autism spectrum disorder*
- Bipolar disorder, including depression and mood instability*
- Augmentation of antidepressants*
- Tourette's disorder*
- Augmentation for treatment-resistant obsessive compulsive disorder
- Second- or third-line treatment for situations involving aggression

There are also many off-label uses for antipsychotics. They may benefit patients with borderline personality traits, eating disorders, and PTSD, usually in small doses. Early indications for chlorpromazine included such nonspecific symptoms as hyperactivity, agitation, anxiety, and "severe behavior," perhaps contributing to over-reliance on this entire class of medications. While antipsychotics can be quite helpful, it's important to remember that they cannot make up for a lack of good therapy or cover for an absence of adult supervision.

CHOOSING ANTIPSYCHOTICS

With all the options available, it can be difficult to decide which antipsychotic to prescribe.

Generally, we recommend avoiding first-generation antipsychotics because of the risk of EPS (extrapyramidal symptoms). We also tend to steer clear of the newest second-generation antipsychotics because they have less of a track record of safety. For these reasons, we favor older second-generation antipsychotics (olanzapine, quetiapine, risperidone, and aripiprazole) over other antipsychotics. Choose specific medications based on side effects, which may be harmful or helpful. If we need to avoid sedation and hunger, we might opt for aripiprazole or risperidone, and if we need to help a person sleep and eat, we might prefer olanzapine or quetiapine. These are rough guidelines as individuals will respond differently.

While new antipsychotics typically come with promises of fewer side effects, we never know much about the real risks until medications are on the market for many years. A recent study reported that in a third of FDA-approved medications, new side effects became apparent only after the agents were approved. If you decide to try a new medication, be sure to include consideration of unknown risks as part of your ongoing process of informed consent.

DISCONTINUING ANTIPSYCHOTICS

When a person responds well to an antipsychotic, we may be tempted to keep it going and make the most of its efficacy, even though there may be little evidence that supports chronic use. On the other hand, we often feel pressed to wean the person off the medication to reduce side effects. Unfortunately, discontinuation often leads to relapse, and relapse often makes recapture of symptoms more difficult. Whatever you decide, think it through and try to go as slowly as practically possible when weaning.

SIDE EFFECTS

1. **Extrapyramidal side effects.** EPS of antipsychotics include dystonia, akathisia, and parkinsonism. Dystonic reactions are painful and frightening. They might include torticollis (twisting neck), opisthotonos (arching back), or oculogyric crisis (eyes rolled back). Tongue swelling can block the airway, causing choking when eating and potentially aspiration pneumonia. Akathisia—severe internal restlessness—can look like overactivity and can create overwhelming anxiety and even suicidality. You may need to use anticholinergics such as benztropine for

dystonia or beta blockers such as propranolol for akathisia. We suggest reviewing EPS as part of informed consent. Although it is rare, you should consider mentioning the symptoms of neuroleptic malignant syndrome. Do a formal screen for signs of tardive dyskinesia (TD) at least every 6 months, eg, with an Abnormal Involuntary Movement Scale (AIMS). (You will find information on conducting the AIMS in the appendices.) Some kids can't cooperate with an AIMS, so you will need to document whatever you are able to see in the office, and perhaps ask parents for home videos if they are reporting new abnormal movements.

2. **Metabolic changes.** Your skinny, out-of-control patient can bloom into a heavy and perhaps still out-of-control patient in a few months. Some people become clinically worse due to their ravenous appetite caused by the medication, becoming more disruptive or devious in their hunt for food. Diet and exercise can be critically important, and we may need to consider switching to less hunger-inducing medications or adding off-label metformin. Both stimulants and topiramate can also mitigate weight gain, although these are off-label uses and must be employed cautiously. Regular metabolic checks are important, including weight and height, calculation of body mass index, fasting lipids and glucose, and perhaps HbA1c and prolactin (with risperidone). Consider checking these labs before treatment, and if they remain normal, at 1, 3, and 6 months, and then annually. Weight gain can also lead to more rapid onset of puberty, with early appearance of secondary sex characteristics and premature closure of growth plates with shorter stature.

3. **Cardiac issues.** Antipsychotics can sometimes create or exacerbate arrhythmias, including QT prolongation with risk for torsades de pointes. Get a good cardiac history and family medical history before starting these medications and consider ordering a screening ECG if there is a significant history of cardiac disease. Some APs, particularly first-generation ones such as chlorpromazine, can also cause orthostatic hypotension.

4. **Prolactin issues.** Some antipsychotics may increase prolactin levels, potentially affecting onset of puberty. Risperidone poses the greatest risk, whereas aripiprazole may have the lowest risk. In patients who present with gynecomastia, prolactin level should be checked. Prolactinemia should also be considered in patients who present with menstrual changes or delayed onset of menarche.

CLASS WARNINGS

All of the second-generation antipsychotics carry the same FDA class warnings. Rather than repeating all of these concerns on each fact sheet, we will mention the warnings here. Some of these are specific to a geriatric population, but we are including them here for completeness.

- In 2003, the FDA required all manufacturers of second-generation antipsychotics to revise their package labeling to reflect the potential risks for weight gain, hyperglycemia, new-onset or worsening diabetes, and hyperlipidemias. While this has become a class warning, it's clear that there are a handful of really bad actors here: Clozapine and olanzapine are the worst, aripiprazole and risperidone relatively less so.

- Patient-specific factors may also play a role. In general, the incidence and severity of weight gain and metabolic effects appear to be greater in the pediatric population.

- A black box warning for all agents in this class suggests a substantially **higher mortality rate in geriatric patients with dementia-related psychosis** receiving second-generation antipsychotics (4.5%) compared with those receiving placebo (2.6%). Although most fatalities resulted from cardiac-related events (eg, heart failure, sudden death) or infections (mostly pneumonia) as opposed to a clearly direct effect of medication, second-generation antipsychotics are *not* approved for the treatment of dementia-related psychosis, and such use should be avoided or minimized when possible.

- **Adverse cerebrovascular events** (eg, stroke, TIA), sometimes fatal, have been reported in geriatric patients (73–97 years of age) with dementia-related psychosis. The FDA has issued a black box warning on second-generation antipsychotics to reflect this risk; several studies have shown that cerebrovascular event risk is elevated with first-generation antipsychotics as well.

- **Neuroleptic malignant syndrome (NMS),** a potentially fatal syndrome characterized by fever, severe muscle rigidity, and autonomic instability, has been reported in patients receiving antipsychotic agents. Treatment requires immediate discontinuation of the drug and intensive symptomatic treatment in a hospital setting.

TABLE 3: First-Generation Antipsychotics

Generic Name (Brand Name) Year FDA Approved [G] denotes generic availability	Relevant FDA Indication(s) (Pediatric indications in bold)	Available Strengths (mg)	Dosage Equivalents	Usual Pediatric Dosage Range (starting–max) (mg)	EPS and Akathisia	Anticholinergic	Relative Sedation and Orthostasis	Notes
Chlorpromazine [G] (Thorazine[1]) 1957	Psychosis, mania, nausea/vomiting; **severe behavioral problems (0.5–17)**; excessive motor activity	10, 25, 50, 100, 200; IM: 25 mg/mL	100	10–200	Low	Moderate	High	Injectable available; photosensitivity
Haloperidol [G] (Haldol, Haldol Decanoate) 1967	**Psychosis (3–17), Tourette's disorder (3–17), severe behavioral problems (3–17)**; excessive motor activity	0.5, 1, 2, 5, 10, 20	2	0.25–10	Very high	Low	Low	Oral solution; injectables (short and LAI) available
Perphenazine [G] (Trilafon[1]) 1957	**Schizophrenia (12 and older)**; severe nausea/vomiting	2, 4, 8, 16	8	8–64	High	Low	Low	Insufficient evidence in kids; mid-potency agent with lower EPS potential than haloperidol

[1] Brand discontinued; no longer available as brand

TABLE 4: Second-Generation Antipsychotics

Generic Name (Brand Name) Year FDA Approved [G] denotes generic availability	Relevant FDA Indication(s) (Pediatric indications in bold)	Available Strengths (mg)	Usual Pediatric Dosage Range (starting–max) (mg)[1]	Weight Gain and Metabolic Effects[2]	EPS and Akathisia	QT Prolongation	Notes
Aripiprazole [G] (Abilify, Abilify Discmelt) 2002	**Schizophrenia (13+), Bipolar mania, monotherapy and adjunctive (10+)**, Bipolar maintenance, monotherapy and adjunctive, Depression adjunct, **Irritability in autism (6–17), Tourette's disorder (6–18)**, Agitation in schizophrenia or bipolar (IM only), Acute schizophrenia relapse (LAI only)	Tablet: 2, 5, 10, 15, 20, 30 ODT: 10, 15 Liquid: 1 mg/mL LAI: Maintena (see fact sheet)	2–30 QD	Moderate	High (mainly akathisia)	Low	Can be "activating"
Asenapine (Saphris) 2009	Schizophrenia, **Bipolar mania, monotherapy and adjunctive (10+)**	Tablet: 2.5, 5, 10 (sublingual only)	5–10 BID	Moderate	Moderate	Low	Avoid food or drink for 10 minutes after taking; sedating
Clozapine [G] (Clozaril, FazaClo, Versacloz) 1989 Generic not available for oral suspension	Treatment-resistant schizophrenia, Recurrent suicidal behavior in schizophrenia or schizoaffective disorders	Tablet: 25, 50, 100, 200 ODT: 12.5, 25, 100, 150, 200 Oral suspension: 50 mg/mL	12.5–450 BID	High	Low	Low	Probably most effective AP, though data in kids limited

Generic Name (Brand Name) Year FDA Approved [G] denotes generic availability	Relevant FDA Indication(s) (Pediatric indications in bold)	Available Strengths (mg)	Usual Pediatric Dosage Range (starting–max) (mg)[1]	Weight Gain and Metabolic Effects[2]	EPS and Akathisia	QT Prolongation	Notes
Lurasidone (Latuda) 2010	**Schizophrenia (13+), bipolar depression (10+)**	Tablet: 20, 40, 60, 80, 120	40–80 QD	Moderate	Moderate	Low	Sedating; must take with food
Olanzapine [G] (Zyprexa, Zyprexa Zydis) 1996 Generic not available for LAI	**Schizophrenia (13+) Bipolar mania, monotherapy and adjunctive (13+)** Bipolar maintenance, monotherapy Agitation in schizophrenia or bipolar (IM only) **Bipolar depression in combination with fluoxetine (10+)**	Tablet: 2.5, 5, 7.5, 10, 15, 20 ODT: 5, 10, 15, 20 IM injection: 10 mg/vial LAI: Relprevv (see fact sheet)	2.5–20 QD	High	Low/moderate	Low	Greatest weight gain, metabolic effects; somnolence
Paliperidone [G] (Invega) 2006 Generic not available for LAI	**Schizophrenia (12+)** Schizoaffective disorder	ER tablet: 1.5, 3, 6, 9 LAI: Sustenna and Trinza (see fact sheet)	3–12 QD	Moderate	High	Moderate	Good for those with hepatic impairment; increases prolactin; fewer data in kids than risperidone
Quetiapine [G] (Seroquel, Seroquel XR) 1997	**Schizophrenia (13+) Bipolar mania, monotherapy and adjunctive (10+)** Bipolar depression Depression adjunct	Tablet: 25, 50, 100, 200, 300, 400 ER tablet: 50, 150, 200, 300, 400	50–800 daily, divided BID to TID; 300–800 QHS for XR	Moderate	Low	Moderate	Sedating; weight gain
Risperidone [G] (Risperdal, Risperdal M-Tab) 1993 Generic not available for LAI	**Schizophrenia (13+) Bipolar mania, monotherapy and adjunctive (10+) Irritability in autism (ages 5–17)**	Tablet: 0.25, 0.5, 1, 2, 3, 4 ODT: 0.25, 0.5, 1, 2, 3, 4 LAI: Consta (see fact sheet)	0.5–6 divided QD to BID	Moderate	High	Low	Increases prolactin; often produces EPS; weight gain
Ziprasidone [G] (Geodon) 2001	Schizophrenia Bipolar mania, monotherapy Bipolar maintenance adjunctive Agitation in schizophrenia (IM injection)	Capsule: 20, 40, 60, 80 IM injection: 20 mg/mL	20–80 BID	Low–moderate	Low	High	Take with food; limited data in kids. Increases prolactin; EPS; weight gain

ODT = orally disintegrating tablet; LAI = long-acting injectable; ER, XR = extended release

[1] For schizophrenia indication

[2] Significant weight gain and metabolic symptoms may occur in kids even with lower-risk agents

ARIPIPRAZOLE (Abilify) Fact Sheet [G]

PEDIATRIC FDA INDICATIONS:
Schizophrenia (13–17 years); **bipolar disorder**, acute treatment of manic and mixed episodes (10–17 years); **irritability in autism** (6–17 years); **Tourette's disorder** (6–18 years).

ADULT FDA INDICATIONS:
Schizophrenia; bipolar disorder, acute treatment of manic and mixed episodes; bipolar disorder, maintenance treatment (adults); major depression, as adjunct.

OFF-LABEL USES:
Bipolar depression; behavioral disturbances.

DOSAGE FORMS:
- **Tablets (G):** 2 mg, 5 mg, 10 mg, 15 mg, 20 mg, 30 mg.
- **Orally disintegrating tablets (G):** 10 mg, 15 mg.
- **Oral liquid (G):** 1 mg/mL.
- **IM depot:** Abilify Maintena: 300 mg and 400 mg; Aristada: 441 mg, 662 mg, 882 mg, 1064 mg (see LAI table).

PEDIATRIC DOSAGE GUIDANCE:
- Schizophrenia and bipolar disorder: Start 2 mg/day, increase on third day to 5 mg/day; may increase further by 5 mg/day increments weekly to target dose 10 mg/day, max 15 mg/day (<11 years) or 30 mg/day (≥12 years).
- Irritability in autism: Start 2 mg/day, increase up to 5 mg/day in weekly increments to target dose 5–10 mg/day, max 15 mg/day.
- Tourette's: Start 2 mg/day, ↑ to target 5 mg/day, max 10 mg/day (<50 kg), 10 mg/day, max 20 mg/day (>50 kg).
- Liquid dosing: Oral solution equivalent to tablet dose up to 25 mg; for 30 mg tablets, give 25 mg oral solution. Generic only.
- Orally disintegrating tablet: Same as regular tablet dosing.

MONITORING: Weight, waist circumference, glucose, lipids, abnormal movements.

COST: $; ODT, liquid: $$$$

SIDE EFFECTS:
- Most common: akathisia, anxiety, insomnia, sedation, tremors, EPS, weight gain.
- Serious but rare: rare reports of reversible pathologic gambling and other impulse control problems (eating, spending, sexual).

MECHANISM, PHARMACOKINETICS, AND DRUG INTERACTIONS:
- Dopamine D2 and serotonin 5HT1A receptor partial agonist and serotonin 5HT2A receptor antagonist.
- Metabolized by CYP450 2D6 and 3A4; t ½: 3–6 days.
- Use ½ usual dose in presence of 2D6 or 3A4 inhibitors or in known 2D6 poor metabolizers; ¼ dose if both 2D6 inhibitor/poor metabolizer and 3A4 inhibitors; double dose if also using 3A4 inducer.

EVIDENCE AND CLINICAL PEARLS:
- A 52-week randomized controlled trial of 146 adolescents with schizophrenia found a longer time to exacerbation of psychotic symptoms and relapse with aripiprazole compared with placebo.
- Aripiprazole is commonly used longer-term in ASD, despite lack of evidence for continued effectiveness.
- One 4-week (n = 296) and one 6-week trial (n = 43) compared aripiprazole with placebo in children with bipolar disorder (and comorbid ADHD in the latter study) and found aripiprazole to be significantly more effective for mania than placebo.
- Two 8-week randomized trials in a total of 308 children (ages 6–17) with autism and irritability showed significant benefit with aripiprazole compared to placebo. In 1 continuation trial of 85 aripiprazole responders who were randomized to either continue aripiprazole or switch to placebo, no difference in time to relapse was seen.
- Several studies have demonstrated aripiprazole's efficacy in reducing tics in children with Tourette's syndrome (significantly more than placebo, as well as equal to risperidone or haloperidol).
- One of 2 FDA-approved medications for irritability in autism. Also, some prescribers use low-dose aripiprazole to counteract antipsychotic-induced prolactinemia, given its partial agonist properties.

FUN FACT:
After aripiprazole's generic launch, Otsuka followed up with brexpiprazole, another dopamine partial agonist, approved for use in adults with schizophrenia and depression (as adjunct) and now in clinical trials for ADHD.

BOTTOM LINE:
Good choice for minimizing risk of weight gain and metabolic side effects, but beware of akathisia. Large number of indications and reports of success at a variety of doses make it difficult to predict dosing for individual patients.

ASENAPINE (Saphris) Fact Sheet

PEDIATRIC FDA INDICATIONS:
Bipolar disorder, acute monotherapy treatment of manic or mixed episodes (10–17 years).

ADULT FDA INDICATIONS:
Schizophrenia; bipolar disorder, acute and maintenance treatment of manic or mixed episodes.

OFF-LABEL USES:
Bipolar maintenance; bipolar depression; behavioral disturbances; impulse control disorders.

DOSAGE FORMS:
SL tablets: 2.5 mg, 5 mg, 10 mg. (Must be taken sublingually because if swallowed, too much medication is metabolized by the liver during first-pass metabolism.)

PEDIATRIC DOSAGE GUIDANCE:
- Bipolar: Start 2.5 mg BID, increase as needed up to 10 mg BID.
- Do not swallow tablets. Avoid food or drink for 10 minutes after taking (they significantly reduce absorption and bioavailability).

MONITORING: Weight, waist circumference, glucose, lipids, BP, abnormal movements.

COST: $$$$$

SIDE EFFECTS:
- Most common: akathisia (seems to be dose-related), oral hypoesthesia (numbing of the tongue or decreased oral sensitivity), somnolence, fatigue, dizziness, increased appetite, EPS, weight gain.
- Serious but rare: hypersensitivity reactions including anaphylaxis, angioedema, low blood pressure, rapid heart rate, swollen tongue, difficulty breathing, wheezing, or rash; orthostatic hypotension and syncope, particularly early in treatment.

MECHANISM, PHARMACOKINETICS, AND DRUG INTERACTIONS:
- Dopamine D2 and serotonin 5HT2A receptor antagonist.
- Metabolized by glucuronidation and CYP1A2; t ½: 24 hours. Inhibitor of 2D6; may double paroxetine levels. Smoking may induce metabolism and may lower levels of asenapine via 1A2 induction; adjust dosing. CYP1A2 inhibitors (eg, fluvoxamine) may increase levels of asenapine; adjust dose.
- Caution with antihypertensive agents and other drugs that can cause additive hypotension or bradycardia.

EVIDENCE AND CLINICAL PEARLS:
- Asenapine was studied in kids 12–17 with schizophrenia and was found to be no better than placebo.
- A 3-week randomized study of 403 children (age 10–17) with bipolar found significantly greater reduction in symptoms with asenapine compared to placebo.
- Has a receptor-binding profile similar to clozapine, although asenapine has very little anticholinergic activity.
- Weight gain does seem to be a problem in many adults, and rates are higher in pediatric patients.
- Pediatric patients more sensitive to dystonia during first few days of treatment with higher initial or faster escalation of dose.
- Contraindicated in patients with severe hepatic impairment due to 7-fold higher drug levels.
- Most useful for patients who don't like swallowing pills.

FUN FACT:
Black cherry flavor developed after patients complained about original tablets.

BOTTOM LINE:
Since there are no clear advantages over other second-generation antipsychotics and minimal evidence for efficacy in children, the only reason to prescribe Saphris is if your patient can't or doesn't want to swallow a pill. Mouth numbness, sedation, dizziness, akathisia, weight gain, and potential for allergic reaction are significant liabilities. Not recommended for first-line use.

CHLORPROMAZINE (Thorazine) Fact Sheet [G]

PEDIATRIC FDA INDICATIONS:
Severe behavioral problems (6 months–17 years); **excessive motor activity and impulsivity.**

ADULT FDA INDICATIONS:
Psychosis; mania; nausea and vomiting; intractable hiccups.

OFF-LABEL USES:
Bipolar disorder; impulse control disorders.

DOSAGE FORMS:
- **Tablets (G):** 10 mg, 25 mg, 50 mg, 100 mg, 200 mg.
- **Injectable (G):** 25 mg/mL.

PEDIATRIC DOSAGE GUIDANCE:
Start 0.5 mg/kg Q4–6 hours PRN (eg, 20 kg or 45 lb child, use 10 mg Q4–6 hours PRN). In more severe patients, doses may range up to 50–100 mg/day or 200 mg/day in older children.

MONITORING: BP/P; ECG in patients at risk; prolactin in patients with symptoms, lipids, glucose, abnormal movements.

COST: $$$

SIDE EFFECTS:
- Most common: sedation, orthostasis, tachycardia, drowsiness, dry mouth, constipation, blurred vision, prolactin elevation (sexual side effects, amenorrhea, galactorrhea), EPS, weight gain.
- Serious but rare: skin pigmentation and ocular changes (both dose related); jaundice.

MECHANISM, PHARMACOKINETICS, AND DRUG INTERACTIONS:
- Dopamine D2 receptor antagonist.
- Metabolized primarily by CYP2D6, also 1A2 and 3A4. Patients who are poor metabolizers of CYP2D6 metabolize the drug more slowly; may have increased effects; t ½: 23–37 hours.
- CYP2D6 inhibitors (eg, fluoxetine, paroxetine, quinidine) may increase chlorpromazine levels.

EVIDENCE AND CLINICAL PEARLS:
- Although used in children (especially those with autism spectrum and related disorders) for many years, data supporting its use are minimal and side effects may be significant.
- While chlorpromazine is approved for treating children with excessive motor activity and impulsivity (symptoms consistent with ADHD), stimulants were found to be more effective than antipsychotics in studies comparing the two.
- Chlorpromazine is a low-potency conventional (first-generation) antipsychotic; this leads to less EPS compared to high-potency agents (eg, haloperidol, fluphenazine) and to more anticholinergic side effects compared to mid- and high-potency agents (eg, perphenazine and haloperidol, respectively).
- Extremely sedating agent and often used for this effect. Dosing limited by orthostasis and sedation.

FUN FACT:
Thorazine was developed by a French surgeon in 1948 to induce relaxation and indifference in surgical patients.

BOTTOM LINE:
Not commonly used in children, but may be considered in those with severe behavioral disturbances who may benefit from sedation.

CLOZAPINE (Clozaril) Fact Sheet [G]

PEDIATRIC FDA INDICATIONS:
None.

ADULT FDA INDICATIONS:
Treatment-resistant schizophrenia; reduction in risk of suicide in schizophrenia and schizoaffective disorder.

OFF-LABEL USES:
Treatment-resistant bipolar disorder; treatment-resistant aggression and violence.

DOSAGE FORMS:
- **Tablets (Clozaril):** 25 mg, 100 mg (scored).
- **Tablets (G):** 25 mg, 50 mg, 100 mg, 200 mg (scored).
- **Orally disintegrating tablets (FazaClo, G):** 12.5 mg, 25 mg, 100 mg, 150 mg, 200 mg.
- **Oral suspension (Versacloz):** 50 mg/mL.

PEDIATRIC DOSAGE GUIDANCE:
- No guidance on dosing in children and adolescents.
- Start 12.5 mg once or twice daily; ↑ gradually, in increments of 25 mg–50 mg/day every few days to response. Max 900 mg/day (adolescents).
- If dosing is interrupted for ≥48 hours, must be re-titrated from 12.5 mg–25 mg/day; may be increased more rapidly than initial titration, as tolerated.

MONITORING: Weight, waist circumference, glucose, lipids, BP/P; ECG in patients at risk, abnormal movements. Clinician must take a brief training course to enroll in REMS and then enroll patient. Before starting clozapine, ensure absolute neutrophil count (ANC) >1500; consult Clozapine REMS (https://www.clozapinerems.com/CpmgClozapineUI/rems/pdf/resources/ANC_Table.pdf) for advice. Serum level monitoring can be useful in adults; minimal guidance for pediatric patients.

COST: $$$; oral suspension, ODT: $$$$$

SIDE EFFECTS:
- Most common: sedation, orthostatic hypotension, hypersalivation (place towel on pillow), weight gain (15–30 pound average weight gain after 1 year), constipation (risk of toxic megacolon if untreated), tachycardia (can treat with propranolol).
- Serious but rare: potentially life-threatening agranulocytosis (1%–2%); periodic WBC testing (as above, see prescribing information for monitoring details) must occur.

MECHANISM, PHARMACOKINETICS, AND DRUG INTERACTIONS:
- Dopamine D2 and serotonin 5HT2A receptor antagonist.
- Metabolized by several CYP450: 1A2, 2D6, and 3A4; t ½: 12 hours.
- Avoid use with drugs that may cause bone marrow suppression (eg, carbamazepine) and lower seizure threshold. Collapse, respiratory arrest, and cardiac arrest reported during initial clozapine treatment in patients taking benzodiazepines. Caution with P450 inhibitors and inducers.

EVIDENCE AND CLINICAL PEARLS:
- Risk of agranulocytosis greatest within first 6 months, then incidence declines but can still occur.
- Divided doses may minimize some adverse effects (eg, hypotension, seizures).
- Limited data from 3 randomized clinical trials in children (as young as 6 years of age) showed better efficacy than haloperidol, olanzapine, and high-dose olanzapine.
- One small retrospective study in adolescents found decreased cannabis use and psychotic symptoms in those with concurrent psychosis and substance use.

FUN FACTS:
The Quiet Room is a compelling memoir written by patient Lori Schiller, who was an early user of clozapine.

BOTTOM LINE:
The only drug with convincing evidence based on years of clinical experience to help treatment-resistant schizophrenia, but only minimal data in children. Consider in severe cases, after failure of other agents.

HALOPERIDOL (Haldol) Fact Sheet [G]

PEDIATRIC FDA INDICATIONS:
Psychosis (3–17 years); **Tourette's syndrome** (3–17 years); **severe behavioral problems** (3–17 years); **excessive motor activity, impulsivity** (3–17 years).

ADULT FDA INDICATIONS:
Psychosis; Tourette's disorder.

OFF-LABEL USES:
Bipolar disorder; impulse control disorders; delirium.

DOSAGE FORMS:
- **Tablets (G):** 0.5 mg, 1 mg, 2 mg, 5 mg, 10 mg, 20 mg (scored).
- **Oral concentrate (G):** 2 mg/mL.
- **Injectable (G):** 5 mg/mL.
- **Depot injection (G):** 50 mg/mL and 100 mg/mL (see LAI fact sheet and table).

PEDIATRIC DOSAGE GUIDANCE:
- Weight-based guideline: 0.05 mg/kg/day–0.2 mg/kg/day.
- Start 0.25 mg–0.5 mg/day; increase by 0.25 mg–0.5 mg increments every 5–7 days and adjust to lowest effective dose; usual range 0.5 mg–5 mg/day, although doses up to 10 mg/day may be used in older children.

MONITORING: Prolactin, glucose, lipids, weight, waist circumference, EPS, abnormal movements.

COST: $

SIDE EFFECTS:
- Most common: EPS, headache, drowsiness, dry mouth, prolactin elevation (sexual side effects, amenorrhea, galactorrhea).
- Serious but rare: See class warnings in chapter introduction.

MECHANISM, PHARMACOKINETICS, AND DRUG INTERACTIONS:
- Dopamine D2 receptor antagonist.
- Metabolized primarily by CYP2D6, also 3A4; t ½: 21–24 hours. Patients that are poor metabolizers of CYP2D6 metabolize the drug more slowly; may have increased effects.
- CYP2D6 inhibitors (eg, fluoxetine, paroxetine, quinidine) may increase haloperidol levels. May inhibit CYP2D6; caution with substrates of 2D6 as haloperidol may increase their levels and effects.

EVIDENCE AND CLINICAL PEARLS:
- Older data in children with Tourette's, severe behavioral disorders, and psychosis show some benefit. Haloperidol is also the most well-studied first-generation antipsychotic in treating children with autism.
- Although haloperidol is approved for treating children with excessive motor activity and impulsivity (symptoms consistent with ADHD), stimulants have been shown to be more effective than antipsychotics in studies comparing the two.
- Haloperidol is a high-potency conventional (first-generation) antipsychotic; this leads to more EPS compared to mid- or low-potency agents (eg, perphenazine or chlorpromazine, respectively) and to less sedation, less orthostasis, and fewer anticholinergic side effects compared to low-potency agents (eg, chlorpromazine).
- Relatively lower seizure side effect risk compared to lower-potency agents.
- Availability of short-acting injectable and oral liquid formulations allows for more flexibility in administration.
- Long-acting injectable decanoate formulation allows option for patients who don't take oral formation reliably.

FUN FACT:
Haldol was discovered in 1958 by Paul Janssen, the founder of Belgian pharmaceutical company Janssen Pharmaceutica.

BOTTOM LINE:
Haloperidol is an effective, inexpensive first-generation antipsychotic with a long history of experience and use even in kids, but clinical utility is limited due to potential for EPS, prolactin elevation, and TD.

LURASIDONE (Latuda) Fact Sheet

PEDIATRIC FDA INDICATIONS:
Schizophrenia (13–17 years); **bipolar depression** (10–17 years).

ADULT FDA INDICATIONS:
Schizophrenia; bipolar depression (as monotherapy and adjunct).

OFF-LABEL USES:
Mixed depression; treatment-resistant depression; manic episodes; impulse control disorders.

DOSAGE FORMS:
Tablets: 20 mg, 40 mg, 60 mg, 80 mg, 120 mg.

PEDIATRIC DOSAGE GUIDANCE:
Start 40 mg QD, with food (at least 350 calories); no titration required. Usual dose 40 mg–80 mg/day. Max dose 80 mg/day for adolescents vs 160 mg/day in adults.

MONITORING: Weight, waist circumference, glucose, lipids, BP/P, abnormal movements.

COST: $$$$$

SIDE EFFECTS:
- Most common: somnolence (dose-related), EPS, akathisia (dose-related), nausea and vomiting, weight gain.
- Serious but rare: orthostatic hypotension and syncope reported (rarely).

MECHANISM, PHARMACOKINETICS, AND DRUG INTERACTIONS:
- Dopamine D2 and serotonin 5HT2A and 5HT7 antagonist; serotonin 5HT1A partial agonist.
- Metabolized primarily through CYP450 3A4; t ½: 18 hours.
- Avoid use with medications that cause orthostasis, potent 3A4 inhibitors (eg, ketoconazole, clarithromycin), or inducers (eg, rifampin, St. John's wort, carbamazepine). Exercise caution/monitor when using in combination with moderate 3A4 inhibitors (eg, diltiazem); decrease lurasidone dose by 50% in patients taking moderate 3A4 inhibitors.

EVIDENCE AND CLINICAL PEARLS:
- Newest indication of bipolar depression in kids is based on a 6-week randomized double-blind placebo-controlled study of 347 kids receiving lurasidone 20–80 mg/day or placebo. Lurasidone-treated patients had a statistically significant larger improvement in symptoms of bipolar depression with an effect size of 0.45 (as measured by Children's Depression Rating Scale, Revised).
- A placebo-controlled study of lurasidone in irritability associated with autism found it no better than placebo, and 13 out of 18 kids between 6–12 years old experienced vomiting.
- Administration with food (at least 350 calories) increases bioavailability 2-fold and peak serum levels roughly 3-fold; fat content of meal is not important.
- Appears to be relatively weight-neutral and cardiometabolic parameters little affected in company-sponsored trials, although post-marketing observations have been limited, particularly in kids.

FUN FACT:
One unique feature of Latuda is its high affinity for the 5-HT7 receptor, which has been linked to depression, learning/memory, cognition, anxiety, and pain. Unfortunately, to date, Latuda has shown no clear benefit over other second-generation antipsychotics on these measures.

BOTTOM LINE:
This drug offers some advantages, including no need for titration, once-daily dosing, relatively low-moderate metabolic profile, and relatively low QTc prolongation risk. However, its use is limited by the need to administer with ≥350 calories of food, potential for drug interactions, and side effects including sedation, akathisia, and EPS, not to mention relatively minimal data (and certainly no long-term data) in kids.

OLANZAPINE (Zyprexa) Fact Sheet [G]

PEDIATRIC FDA INDICATIONS:
Schizophrenia (13–17 years); **bipolar acute mania** (13–17 years); **bipolar depression** (with fluoxetine, as Symbyax, 10–17 years).

ADULT FDA INDICATIONS:
Schizophrenia; acute or mixed bipolar I manic episodes, as monotherapy or adjunct; maintenance treatment of bipolar disorder; bipolar depression (with fluoxetine, as Symbyax); treatment-resistant unipolar depression (with fluoxetine); acute agitation in schizophrenia and bipolar mania (injectable form).

OFF-LABEL USES:
Behavioral disturbances; impulse control disorders.

DOSAGE FORMS:
- **Tablets (G):** 2.5 mg, 5 mg, 7.5 mg, 10 mg, 15 mg, 20 mg.
- **Orally disintegrating tablets (G):** 5 mg, 10 mg, 15 mg, 20 mg.
- **IM injection (G):** 10 mg.
- **Depot injection:** 210 mg, 300 mg, 405 mg (see LAI fact sheet and table).
- **Fixed combination capsules with fluoxetine (G):** 3/25 mg, 6/25 mg, 12/25 mg, 6/50 mg, 12/50 mg olanzapine/fluoxetine.

PEDIATRIC DOSAGE GUIDANCE:
- Schizophrenia and acute mania: Start most at 2.5 mg–5 mg QD, may ↑ by 5 mg QD, in weekly increments, to target dose 10 mg QD; max 20 mg QD.
- Bipolar depression (Symbyax, fixed combination with fluoxetine): Start 3/25 mg QPM, ↑ as indicated to target dose 6 mg/25 mg olanzapine/fluoxetine; max dose 12 mg/50 mg.

MONITORING: Weight, waist circumference, glucose, lipids, abnormal movements.

COST: $; ODT: $$; combination with fluoxetine: $$$

SIDE EFFECTS:
- Most common: somnolence (dose-related), dry mouth (dose-related), constipation, weight gain (up to 40% incidence; may be substantial; 10–30 pounds weight gain is common), increased appetite, EPS (dose-related); increased LFTs; increased prolactin.
- Serious but rare: rare but potentially fatal drug reaction with eosinophilia and systemic symptoms (DRESS) possible; often starting as rash that may spread, fever, swollen lymph nodes, and elevated eosinophils.

MECHANISM, PHARMACOKINETICS, AND DRUG INTERACTIONS:
- Dopamine D2 and serotonin 5HT2A receptor antagonist.
- Metabolized by CYP 450 1A2, 2D6 (minor), and direct glucuronidation; t ½: 1–2 days.
- CYP1A2 inducers (eg, carbamazepine, ritonavir, smoking) may reduce olanzapine levels by 50%; CYP1A2 inhibitors (eg, fluvoxamine) may increase olanzapine bioavailability by 50–100%. Adjust olanzapine dosing in presence of 1A2 inducers or inhibitors.

EVIDENCE AND CLINICAL PEARLS:
Compared to adults, children and adolescents are more likely to gain more weight, experience greater sedation, and have greater increases in LDL cholesterol, total cholesterol, triglycerides, prolactin, and liver transaminase levels.

FUN FACT:
Olanzapine has been studied and is used for chemotherapy-induced nausea and vomiting.

BOTTOM LINE:
Its high risk for weight gain and metabolic complications make it a second-line choice for kids and adolescents.

PALIPERIDONE (Invega) Fact Sheet [G]

PEDIATRIC FDA INDICATIONS:
Schizophrenia (12–17 years).

ADULT FDA INDICATIONS:
Schizophrenia; schizoaffective disorder.

OFF-LABEL USES:
Bipolar disorder; behavioral disturbances; impulse control disorders.

DOSAGE FORMS:
- **Controlled release tablets (G):** 1.5 mg, 3 mg, 6 mg, 9 mg (not breakable).
- **Monthly depot injection (Invega Sustenna):** 39 mg, 78 mg, 117 mg, 156 mg, and 234 mg (see LAI fact sheet and table).
- **Every-3-month depot injection (Invega Trinza):** 273 mg, 410 mg, 546 mg, 819 mg (see LAI fact sheet and table).

PEDIATRIC DOSAGE GUIDANCE:
- Start 3 mg QAM, which may be the effective dose; if required, may ↑ by 3 mg/day at intervals of >5 days to max 6 mg/day (weight <51 kg) or 12 mg/day (weight ≥51 kg).
- Paliperidone 3 mg, 6 mg, 9 mg, and 12 mg roughly equivalent to 1–2 mg, 2–4 mg, 4–6 mg, and 6–8 mg risperidone, respectively.

MONITORING: Weight, waist circumference, glucose, lipids, abnormal movements.

COST: $$$$

SIDE EFFECTS:
- Most common: akathisia, EPS (dose-related), tremor, tachycardia, somnolence, weight gain, prolactin elevation.
- Serious but rare: increase in QTc interval. Orthostatic hypotension and syncope reported. Controlled release tablet may cause GI obstruction in patients with strictures (either pathologic or iatrogenic). Esophageal dysmotility and aspiration possible; use caution in patients at risk for aspiration pneumonia (eg, those with advanced Alzheimer's dementia).

MECHANISM, PHARMACOKINETICS, AND DRUG INTERACTIONS:
- Dopamine D2 and serotonin 5HT2A receptor antagonist.
- Not metabolized by liver; t ½: 23 hours.
- Avoid use with drugs known to prolong the QT interval or to cause orthostasis. Paliperidone is the principal active metabolite of risperidone; therefore, avoid use with risperidone. Minimal drug interactions.

EVIDENCE AND CLINICAL PEARLS:
- An 8-week double-blind randomized trial in 228 adolescents with schizophrenia, with a maintenance period of 18 weeks, found paliperidone was equally effective as aripiprazole.
- An 8-week observational study in 15 kids with mania reported remission in 47% of patients treated with paliperidone.
- An open-label study in kids with autism suggested efficacy.
- Warn your patients that they may find capsules in their stool. These are empty "ghost pills." Invega (and Concerta; see fact sheet) is an extended release tablet based on the OROS osmotic delivery system, which releases medication from a hard shell.
- Swallow whole, with fluids; do not chew, divide, or crush.
- In adult studies, paliperidone is not effective in acute mania even with lithium or valproate.
- Along with risperidone, causes the most EPS and hyperprolactinemia of all the second-generations.

FUN FACT:
First drug with FDA approval for schizoaffective disorder in adults, allowing Janssen to carve out a new marketing niche and separate this drug from its competitors (at least from a commercial and marketing perspective).

BOTTOM LINE:
Invega looks like risperidone without drug-drug interactions, but with more QT interval prolongation, more tachycardia, possibly more EPS, and the same amount of hyperprolactinemia. These significant disadvantages, and relatively fewer data in kids, make it a second-line option.

PERPHENAZINE (Trilafon) Fact Sheet [G]

PEDIATRIC FDA INDICATIONS:
Schizophrenia (12+ years).

ADULT FDA INDICATIONS:
Schizophrenia; severe nausea and vomiting.

OFF-LABEL USES:
Bipolar disorder; behavioral disturbances; impulse control disorders.

DOSAGE FORMS:
Tablets (G): 2 mg, 4 mg, 8 mg, 16 mg.

PEDIATRIC DOSAGE GUIDANCE:
Ages >12: Start 4 mg BID; adjust to lowest effective dose. Dose range 8 mg–16 mg BID–QID; max FDA-approved dose for non-hospitalized patients is 24 mg/day, but hospitalized psychotic patients may be dosed up to 64 mg/day (adults).

MONITORING: Prolactin, lipids, glucose, EPS, abnormal movements.

COST: $$

SIDE EFFECTS:
- Most common: EPS, headache, drowsiness, dry mouth, prolactin elevation (sexual side effects, amenorrhea, galactorrhea).
- Serious but rare: tachycardia (especially with sudden marked increase in dose).

MECHANISM, PHARMACOKINETICS, AND DRUG INTERACTIONS:
- Dopamine D2 receptor antagonist.
- Metabolized primarily by CYP2D6; t ½: 9–12 hours. May inhibit CYP2D6. Poor metabolizers of CYP2D6 metabolize the drug more slowly; may have increased effects.
- CYP2D6 inhibitors (eg, fluoxetine, paroxetine, quinidine) may increase perphenazine levels. Caution with substrates of 2D6 as perphenazine may increase their levels and effects.

EVIDENCE AND CLINICAL PEARLS:
- No clinical trial data in children or adolescents with schizophrenia, but FDA-indicated and used in kids by some clinicians based on experience as well as results from efficacy studies in adults.
- Based on 18-month, randomized trial of 1,493 adult patients with schizophrenia (CATIE trial), perphenazine appears similar in efficacy and EPS compared to second-generation antipsychotics (olanzapine, quetiapine, risperidone, ziprasidone).
- Perphenazine is an intermediate-potency conventional (first-generation) antipsychotic; this leads to less EPS compared to high-potency agents (eg, haloperidol, fluphenazine) and to less sedation, less orthostasis, and fewer anticholinergic side effects compared to low-potency agents (eg, chlorpromazine).
- Fewer metabolic effects (weight gain, glucose, lipids) than some antipsychotics.

FUN FACT:
Perphenazine has long been available in a formulation with amitriptyline (a tricyclic antidepressant) called Triavil. This combination antipsychotic/antidepressant was first available in 1965, foreshadowing the next such combination drug (Symbyax) by 38 years.

BOTTOM LINE:
Well-tolerated and inexpensive alternative to second-generation antipsychotics, especially when trying to avoid EPS and metabolic side effects; however, efficacy data in kids is more limited compared to newer agents.

QUETIAPINE (Seroquel) Fact Sheet [G]

PEDIATRIC FDA INDICATIONS:
Schizophrenia (13–17 years); **bipolar mania** (10–17 years).

ADULT FDA INDICATIONS:
Schizophrenia; bipolar, manic/mixed; bipolar depression; maintenance treatment for bipolar; major depression, as adjunct.

OFF-LABEL USES:
Insomnia; anxiety disorders; behavioral disturbances; impulse control disorders.

DOSAGE FORMS:
- **Tablets (G):** 25 mg, 50 mg, 100 mg, 200 mg, 300 mg, 400 mg.
- **ER tablets (G):** 50 mg, 150 mg, 200 mg, 300 mg, 400 mg.

PEDIATRIC DOSAGE GUIDANCE:
- Adolescents: Start 25 mg BID or 50 mg XR QHS, ↑ dose by 50 mg–100 mg/day increments, every 1–4 days to target/max dose 400–600 mg/day (mania) or 400–800 mg/day (schizophrenia).
- Max dose for <9 years: 400 mg/day.

MONITORING: Prolactin, lipids, glucose, BP, weight, waist circumference, abnormal movements.

COST: IR: $; ER: $$$$

SIDE EFFECTS:
- Most common: somnolence, hypotension, dry mouth, dizziness, weight gain, increased appetite, fatigue, nausea, vomiting, tachycardia, EPS, abnormal movements.
- Serious but rare: Increases in BP occurred in pediatric studies vs orthostasis in adults (15% had systolic elevation >20 mmHg and 40% had diastolic elevation >10 mmHg).

MECHANISM, PHARMACOKINETICS, AND DRUG INTERACTIONS:
- Dopamine D2 and serotonin 5HT2A receptor antagonist.
- Metabolized by CYP3A4; t ½: 6 hours (XR: 7 hours).
- Avoid or use caution with agents that may cause additional orthostasis. CYP3A4 inducers (eg, carbamazepine) may lower quetiapine levels; CYP3A4 inhibitors (eg, erythromycin, ketoconazole) may increase quetiapine levels. Adjust quetiapine dose in presence of CYP3A4 inducers or inhibitors.

EVIDENCE AND CLINICAL PEARLS:
- A 6-week randomized controlled trial in 220 adolescents with schizophrenia found quetiapine was significantly more effective than placebo at reducing psychotic symptoms.
- A 3-week randomized trial in 277 kids (ages 10–17) with bipolar disorder found significantly higher remission rates with quetiapine compared to placebo.
- A 4-week randomized trial in 50 kids (ages 12–18) with bipolar disorder found significantly higher remission rates with quetiapine than divalproex.
- A study in bipolar depression in kids ages 10–17 did not find quetiapine XR more effective than placebo. Two open-label studies in autism did not find it to be effective either.
- Swallow XR tablet whole; do not break, crush, or chew; switch between IR and XR at the same total daily dose; dose adjustments may be necessary based on response and tolerability.
- If patient discontinues drug >1 week, re-titrate dose as with initial therapy.
- Quetiapine abuse has been reported, particularly in incarcerated adult populations.
- Nearly 20% of children gained >7% of body weight (adjusted for usual growth) after 26 weeks of quetiapine.

FUN FACT:
Cataracts developed in initial studies with beagle dogs; human studies have not shown an association. However, the label still recommends a slit-lamp exam every 6 months.

BOTTOM LINE:
Lower risk for EPS and a broad spectrum of efficacy make this an appealing first-choice agent. However, sedation, weight gain, and orthostasis may limit use. Dosing at bedtime, or switching to XR, may help reduce daytime sedation.

RISPERIDONE (Risperdal) Fact Sheet [G]

PEDIATRIC FDA INDICATIONS:
Schizophrenia (13–17 years); **bipolar mania, monotherapy and adjunctive** (10–17 years); **irritability in autism** (5–17 years).

ADULT FDA INDICATIONS:
Schizophrenia; bipolar disorder, manic/mixed.

OFF-LABEL USES:
Bipolar depression; behavioral disturbances; impulse control disorders; Tourette's syndrome.

DOSAGE FORMS:
- **Tablets (G):** 0.25 mg, 0.5 mg, 1 mg, 2 mg, 3 mg, 4 mg.
- **Oral solution (G):** 1 mg/mL.
- **Orally disintegrating tablets (Risperdal M-Tab, G):** 0.25 mg, 0.5 mg, 1 mg, 2 mg, 3 mg, 4 mg.
- **Depot injection (Risperdal Consta):** 12.5 mg, 25 mg, 37.5 mg, 50 mg (see LAI fact sheet and table).

PEDIATRIC DOSAGE GUIDANCE:
- Autism (children ≥5 years): If <15 kg (33 lbs), use with caution. For 15 kg–20 kg (33 lbs–44 lbs), start 0.25 mg/day, ↑ to 0.5 mg/day after ≥4 days. If response insufficient, may ↑ by 0.25 mg/day in ≥2-week intervals; give QD or BID. For ≥20 kg (44 lbs), start 0.5 mg/day; may ↑ to 1 mg/day after ≥4 days. If response insufficient, may ↑ dose by 0.5 mg/day in ≥2-week intervals; give QD or BID.
- Bipolar mania or schizophrenia (children): Start 0.5 mg QD; ↑ in increments of 0.5 mg–1 mg/day at intervals ≥24 hours to target dose of 2 mg–3 mg/day; doses >3 mg/day do not confer additional benefit and are associated with increased side effects.

MONITORING: Weight, waist circumference, glucose, lipids, BP; prolactin, abnormal movements.

COST: $; ODT: $$–$$$ (depending on dose)

SIDE EFFECTS:
- Most common: EPS, somnolence, anxiety, dizziness, salivary hypersecretion, fatigue, prolactin elevation, weight gain, increased appetite.
- Serious but rare: Orthostatic hypotension may occur, particularly at higher doses or with rapid titration. Hyperprolactinemia with clinical symptoms (sexual side effects, galactorrhea, amenorrhea).

MECHANISM, PHARMACOKINETICS, AND DRUG INTERACTIONS:
- Dopamine D2 and serotonin 5HT2A receptor antagonist.
- Metabolized by CYP2D6; t ½: 20 hours.
- CYP2D6 inhibitors (eg, fluoxetine, paroxetine, quinidine) may increase effects of risperidone; reduce risperidone dose. Carbamazepine reduces levels and effects of risperidone; may need to double risperidone dose.

EVIDENCE AND CLINICAL PEARLS:
- Seven published trials have reported efficacy of risperidone in adolescents with schizophrenia (2 open-label, 2 comparisons with olanzapine and haloperidol, 2 comparisons with olanzapine, and 1 randomized placebo-controlled study).
- A 3-week randomized trial in 169 children (ages 10–17) with bipolar mania found significantly higher remission rates with risperidone compared to placebo. A 6-week randomized trial in 66 kids (ages 8–18) with bipolar mania found significantly higher remission rates with risperidone compared to divalproex. An 8-week open-label trial in 279 kids (ages 6–15) with bipolar mania found higher response rates with risperidone compared to both lithium and divalproex sodium; responses to lithium vs divalproex were similar.
- In kids with autism, associated irritability as well as symptoms of aggression towards others, deliberate self-injuriousness, temper tantrums, and quickly changing moods are improved.
- In studies with kids, about 1/3 gained more than 7% of body weight, and over 80% had elevations in prolactin (dose-related, more frequent in girls than boys).
- Along with paliperidone, causes the most EPS and hyperprolactinemia of all the second-generation antipsychotics.
- When reinitiating after discontinuation, initial titration schedule should be followed.

FUN FACT:
Risperdal M-tabs are marketed in other countries as Risperdal Quicklets.

BOTTOM LINE:
Risperidone offers more efficacy and safety data in kids than other antipsychotics and is often used first-line in kids with autism. Monitor carefully for EPS, prolactin, and weight gain.

ZIPRASIDONE (Geodon) Fact Sheet [G]

PEDIATRIC FDA INDICATIONS:
None.

ADULT FDA INDICATIONS:
Schizophrenia; bipolar disorder, acute treatment of manic/mixed episode; maintenance treatment of bipolar disorder as adjunct; acute agitation in patients with schizophrenia (IM only).

OFF-LABEL USES:
Bipolar disorder; behavioral disturbances; impulse control disorders; Tourette's disorder.

DOSAGE FORMS:
- **Capsules (G):** 20 mg, 40 mg, 60 mg, 80 mg.
- **Injection (Geodon):** 20 mg/mL.

PEDIATRIC DOSAGE GUIDANCE:
- No guidance on dosing in children and adolescents.
- Schizophrenia, bipolar disorder: Start 20 mg BID (40 mg BID for acute mania) with meals for 2–3 days; ↑ by 40 mg/day increments; can usually ↑ rather quickly to target dose 60 mg–80 mg BID. Max approved dose is 160 mg/day, though can go higher in some patients; there are some safety data for doses up to 320 mg/day.
- Schizophrenia, acute agitation (IM injection): 10 mg Q2 hours or 20 mg Q4 hours; max 40 mg/day. Replace with oral therapy as soon as possible.

MONITORING: Weight, waist circumference, glucose, lipids; ECG, abnormal movements.

COST: $

SIDE EFFECTS:
- Most common: somnolence, dizziness, akathisia, rash (5%), weight gain, EPS, abnormal movements.
- Serious but rare: May result in minor QTc prolongation (dose-related; 10 msec at 160 mg/day). Clinically relevant prolongation (>500 msec) rare (0.06%) and less than placebo (0.23%). Significant QTc prolongation has been associated with the development of malignant ventricular arrhythmias (torsades de pointes) and sudden death. Avoid in patients with hypokalemia, hypomagnesemia, bradycardia, persistent QTc intervals >500 msec, or those receiving other drugs that prolong QTc interval. Patients with symptoms of dizziness, palpitations, or syncope should receive further cardiac evaluation. Drug reaction with eosinophilia and systemic symptoms (DRESS) has been reported with ziprasidone exposure. DRESS begins as a rash that can spread all over the body; it may include swollen lymph nodes, fever, and damage to organs such as the heart, liver, pancreas, or kidneys, and is sometimes fatal. Discontinue ziprasidone if DRESS is suspected.

MECHANISM, PHARMACOKINETICS, AND DRUG INTERACTIONS:
- Dopamine D2 and serotonin 5HT2A receptor antagonist.
- Metabolized in liver principally by aldehyde oxidase; less than one-third of clearance mediated by CYP450: CYP3A4 (major), and CYP1A2 (minor); t ½: 7 hours.
- Avoid use with other drugs that prolong QTc interval.

EVIDENCE AND CLINICAL PEARLS:
- One 6-week (with 26-week open-label extension) placebo-controlled randomized trial in adolescents with schizophrenia failed to show separation between ziprasidone and placebo in efficacy measures.
- A 4-week randomized trial in 237 children and adolescents (ages 10–17) found significantly greater symptom reduction and response rates with ziprasidone compared to placebo.
- Only limited data with ziprasidone in kids with autism spectrum disorder or Tourette's.
- Administer twice daily, ideally with meals; ingestion of several hundred calories is necessary to increase absorption up to 2-fold.
- Causes less weight gain than clozapine, olanzapine, quetiapine, or risperidone.
- Average increase in QTc greater than any other second-generations, although not much more than for quetiapine. Post-marketing surveillance has shown one or two instances of torsades de pointes possibly related to ziprasidone use.

FUN FACT:
The brand name Geodon has been suggested to bring to mind the phrase "down (don) to earth (geo)," referring to the goals of the medication.

BOTTOM LINE:
Minimal efficacy and safety data in kids, along with disadvantages including twice-daily dosing, need to administer with food, and relatively great QT prolongation, deter us from using this in our pediatric patients.

LONG-ACTING INJECTABLE (LAI) Antipsychotics

INTRODUCTION: IS THERE A ROLE FOR LAIS IN CHILDREN AND ADOLESCENTS?
LAIs are sometimes used for children and adolescents who need antipsychotics for severe illness, but who have difficulty consistently taking oral meds. A 2017 literature review found a few case series and case reports on such children, including a total of 36 individuals with a mean age of about 12. Most were boys, the most common diagnosis was bipolar disorder, and the majority of patients were on either risperidone or paliperidone palmitate. Most of these kids improved on the LAI, and weight gain was the most common side effect (https://tinyurl.com/yb4wq5zb).

Much more research is available for adults, and while results are mixed, in naturalistic studies that focus on real-world patients who are most likely to be prescribed LAIs (that is, those who have a history of non-adherence), it's clear that switching to injectables decreases the risk of hospitalization (Kishimoto T et al, *J Clin Psychiatry* 2013;74(10):957–965).

DECIDING AMONG THE LAIS
General notes on LAIs
- It's best to choose an LAI version of an oral medication that your patient has already taken, so that you can be more confident that the agent is effective and tolerable.
- Be patient; full therapeutic effect of LAIs take longer than orals—ie, several months. Don't adjust the dose prematurely.
- Consider oral overlap. Agents differ on how quickly you can titrate up the dose. This is important because patients requiring gradual titration will need oral pills to make sure they have a decent serum level right away. This process is called the "oral overlap," and it has two disadvantages. First, it makes the process of dosing a bit more complex (not a huge deal); second, if the patient is refusing to take oral meds (but accepting an injection, either under court order or voluntarily), you'll have to choose a different LAI or risk a decompensation while waiting for levels to become therapeutic.
- *Never* initiate an LAI on a patient who has a history of neuroleptic malignant syndrome (NMS) on any antipsychotic. That's just asking for trouble.

LAI options
There's a pretty comprehensive table on the following pages that reports, for each LAI, the **FDA indication(s), medication names, costs, available strengths, dosing information,** and **pharmacokinetics** (need for oral overlap and dosing interval). But first, we'll give you a shorthand version of the most clinically relevant **clinical pearls** below:

First-generation antipsychotics
- **Fluphenazine (Prolixin Decanoate)**—Dosed every 2 weeks. Injections are painful. Cheap, but relatively high risk of EPS and TD. Oral overlap required.
- **Haloperidol (Haldol Decanoate)**—Dosed monthly. As cheap as Prolixin, and since it's dosed less often and the pharmacokinetics are more predictable, it's generally the better choice among FGAs. Oral overlap required, although some use a "loading dose" method (20 times oral dose, followed by 10–15 times oral dose in subsequent months) that requires no oral overlap (Ereshefsky L et al, *Hosp Community Psychiatry* 1993;44(12):1155–1161).

Second-generation antipsychotics
- **Aripiprazole (Abilify Maintena)**—Dosed monthly. Oral overlap required for 14 days. Deltoid or gluteal injection. Expensive. Good side effect profile.
- **Aripiprazole lauroxil (Aristada)**—Dosed monthly, every 6 weeks, or every 2 months. Smallest dose (441 mg monthly) may be given deltoid or gluteal; other doses must be given gluteal. Dosing interval flexibility makes this formulation appealing, although oral overlap is required for 21 days. Expensive. Good side effect profile.
- **Olanzapine (Zyprexa Relprevv)**—Dosed either every 2 weeks or monthly, depending on the dose needed. May be the worst choice among all LAIs for multiple reasons. High potential for weight gain. There's a small risk of a post-injection delirium/sedation syndrome, occurring in less than 1% of patients, caused by accidental intravascular injection. For this reason, you have to give the injection at a registered health care facility where patients can be continuously monitored for at least 3 hours after the injection. Restricted use requires physician and facility registration, and additional paperwork with Eli Lilly's program. High cost, restriction of use, monitoring requirement, and risk of adverse outcome all limit use severely. Gluteal injection only. Expensive. No oral overlap.
- **Paliperidone palmitate monthly (Invega Sustenna)**—Monthly dosing. Less painful injection than Risperdal Consta or Zyprexa Relprevv. No oral overlap required; need for 2 separate loading injections makes initiation a bit more complicated. First 2 doses deltoid; subsequent doses may be deltoid or gluteal. Expensive. No oral overlap and potential to transition to every-3-month formulation are appealing features.
- **Paliperidone palmitate every 3 months (Invega Trinza)**—Every-3-month dosing, but your patient must have done well on monthly injections of Sustenna for at least 4 months before switching to Trinza. Deltoid or gluteal injection. Must shake syringe vigorously for at least 15 seconds to ensure uniform suspension of long-acting particles and prevent clogging in needle. Expensive. No oral overlap.
- **Risperidone (Risperdal Consta)**—Every-2-week dosing; 3-week oral overlap. Cumbersome; must be refrigerated and shaken for at least 10 seconds. Painful deltoid or gluteal. Expensive.

TABLE 5: Long-Acting Injectable (LAI) Antipsychotics

Generic Name (Brand Name) Year FDA Approved [G] denotes generic availability	Relevant FDA Indication(s)	Available Strengths	Oral Overlap	Dosing Interval	Initial Dosing	Maintenance Dose	Cost for Monthly Supply at Average Dose (May 2018)
First-Generation Antipsychotics							
Fluphenazine decanoate [G] (Prolixin Decanoate¹) 1972	Schizophrenia	25 mg/mL	Continue total oral dose for 2–3 days, then ↓ by 50% increments every 2–3 days until discontinued (by next injection)	2 weeks	1.25 X total daily oral dose Q2–3 weeks (5–11 yrs: 3.125 mg–12.5 mg; ≥12 yrs: 6.25 mg–25 mg)	Increase in increments of 3.125 mg–12.5 mg; do not exceed 25 mg per dose	$ [G]
Haloperidol decanoate [G] (Haldol Decanoate) 1986	Schizophrenia	50 mg/mL and 100 mg/mL	For 7 days, give usual oral dose, then ↓ by 50% weekly for 2 weeks, then discontinue	4 weeks	10–20 X total oral daily dose Q4 weeks. First dose should be ≤100 mg; if higher dose needed, give remainder in 1–2 weeks.	Lower to 10–15 X total oral daily dose Q4 weeks	$ [G] $$$$ Haldol Dec
Second-Generation Antipsychotics							
Aripiprazole (Abilify Maintena) 2013	Schizophrenia	300 mg and 400 mg vials	For 14 days	4 weeks	400 mg Q4 weeks	400 mg Q4 weeks; decrease to 300 mg Q4 weeks if side effects	$$$$$
Aripiprazole lauroxil (Aristada) 2015	Schizophrenia	441 mg, 662 mg, 882 mg, 1064 mg	For 21 days	Monthly, every 6 weeks, or every 2 months	441 mg, 662 mg, or 882 mg monthly (equiv to 10, 15, and 20 mg/day); or 882 mg every 6 weeks (15 mg/day); or 1064 mg every 2 months (15 mg/day)	Continue initial dosing or adjust based on clinical response	$$$$$
Olanzapine (Zyprexa Relprevv) 2009	Schizophrenia	210, 300, and 405 mg vials	No overlap	2–4 weeks	10 mg/day oral: 210 mg Q2 weeks x 4 doses or 405 mg Q4 weeks x 2 doses; 15 mg/day oral: 300 mg Q2 weeks x 4 doses; 20 mg/day oral: 300 mg Q2 weeks	10 mg/day oral: 150 mg Q2 weeks or 300 mg Q4 weeks; 15 mg/day oral: 210 mg Q2 weeks or 405 mg Q4 weeks; 20 mg/day oral: 300 mg Q2 weeks; Maximum dose: 300 mg Q2 weeks or 405 mg Q4 weeks	$$$$$
Paliperidone palmitate (Invega Sustenna) 2009	Schizophrenia Schizoaffective disorder (monotherapy or adjunct)	39, 78, 117, 156, and 234 mg in prefilled syringes	No overlap	4 weeks	234 mg IM in deltoid, then 156 mg 1 week later	117 mg 3 weeks after 2nd dose then Q month; may adjust monthly dose (maintenance given deltoid or gluteal) Approx. equivalence: 3 mg oral: 39 mg–78 mg 6 mg oral: 117 mg 12 mg oral: 234 mg	$$$$$

Generic Name (Brand Name) Year FDA Approved [G] denotes generic availability	Relevant FDA Indication(s)	Available Strengths	Oral Overlap	Dosing Interval	Initial Dosing	Maintenance Dose	Cost for Monthly Supply at Average Dose (May 2018)
Paliperidone palmitate (Invega Trinza) 2015	Schizophrenia (only after at least 4 months of adequate treatment on Invega Sustenna)	273, 410, 546, 819 mg in prefilled syringes	No overlap	3 months	Based on previous Invega Sustenna dose: • for 78 mg, give 273 mg Trinza • for 117 mg, give 410 mg Trinza • for 156 mg, give 546 mg Trinza • for 234 mg, give 819 mg Trinza	Give same conversion dose of Trinza every 3 months; adjust if necessary per patient response	$$$$$
Risperidone (Risperdal Consta)† 2003	Schizophrenia Bipolar, manic/mixed (monotherapy or adjunct)	12.5, 25, 37.5, and 50 mg vials	With usual oral dose for 3 weeks	2 weeks	Start at 25 mg Q2 weeks. Adjust dose no more frequently than Q4 weeks as needed for response.	Approx. equivalence: <4 mg/day oral: 25 mg 4 mg–6 mg/day oral: 37.5 mg >6 mg/day oral: 50 mg Maximum dose: 50 mg Q2 weeks	$$$$$

†brand discontinued; available as generic only

Anxiolytics and Hypnotics

ANXIOLYTICS

Anxiety is perhaps the most frequent symptom for which child psychiatrists are consulted. There are many medications to choose from, and clinicians all have their personal algorithms, which will vary depending on the clinical situation. While SSRIs are generally considered the mainstay medications for anxiety, it is important to consider other options, particularly because of SSRIs' potential for side effects. Here are some pros and cons of the major options.

Alpha adrenergics: Central alpha agonists include the alpha-2 agonists guanfacine and clonidine, plus the alpha-1 antagonist prazosin. These medications are approved for use in hypertension, and some of them are approved for ADHD. They reduce sympathetic tone, resulting in a mild reduction in internal tension and vigilance that is often very helpful. They are also useful in reducing tics. Prazosin can be helpful for nightmares, particularly those associated with PTSD. Common side effects include dizziness and sedation. These medications often have associated tachyphylaxis (ie, rapid tolerance to the dose, resulting in a need for higher dose); however, this tends to abate after the first few weeks. Central alpha agonists are associated with irritability, perhaps related to the sedation they create.

Beta blockers: The most commonly used beta blocker in child psychiatry is propranolol. It is useful for performance anxiety and other situations in which reducing the physiological symptoms of anxiety (ie, rapid or pounding heartbeat) would be helpful. There has been recent interest in using propranolol to help children with autism become more comfortable with social situations. Common side effects include reduced blood pressure in teens and reduced exercise tolerance in children and teens. Of note, fluoxetine can increase levels of propranolol, and if this leads to more tiredness, it may be mistaken as depression and lead to an unnecessary increase of the fluoxetine dose.

SSRIs: SSRIs are the only FDA-approved medications for anxiety disorders in children, specifically fluoxetine, fluvoxamine, and sertraline for obsessive-compulsive disorder (OCD). Beyond OCD, SSRIs have a broad research evidence base for anxiety in children and adolescents, including studies in generalized anxiety disorder (GAD), social phobia, and separation anxiety. In general, we recommend using a lower initial dose of SSRI for patients with anxiety disorders, particularly panic disorder. The disadvantage of SSRIs is their substantial side effects, in particular behavioral activation, which can be mistaken for increased anxiety, ADHD, or oppositionality. Like adults, children and teens may also experience side effects such as amotivational syndrome, manic or hypomanic episodes, GI disturbances, and excessive sweating (the latter a possible harbinger of a hyperserotonergic syndrome).

Mirtazapine: Mirtazapine is helpful for anxiety, depression, insomnia, poor appetite, and gastrointestinal distress in adults. It may be appropriate for some kids, though pediatric data are mostly limited to kids with depression. Side effects include sedation and overeating.

SNRIs: Except for OCD, for which SNRIs have less utility, these medications have similar uses as SSRIs. A distinct disadvantage of SNRIs is their tendency toward problems with physiological withdrawal. Of the SNRIs, duloxetine is the only agent with an FDA indication for GAD (for kids 7 and up). Venlafaxine showed superiority over placebo in studies of kids with social anxiety and GAD.

Buspirone: Buspirone may have some value in some children and teens with anxiety symptoms. While there are case reports of efficacy, there is 1 negative study for GAD. Buspirone may help in GAD, but it's unlikely to help in other anxiety disorders. It is relatively innocuous in terms of side effects and may be worth trying in a patient with generalized anxiety.

Tricyclic antidepressants (TCA): In former days, TCAs were considered a panacea for children's "behavioral issues," used for anxiety, depression, insomnia, ADHD, and bedwetting. Concerns about cardiac dangers dampened enthusiasm; however, clomipramine remains frequently used for OCD when SSRIs or SNRIs fail. In addition, neurologists and others continue to use TCAs for migraine and other pain syndromes. ECGs are recommended at initiation and follow-up due to risks of arrhythmias, including the potentially deadly torsades de pointes. These medications must be kept securely locked away as they are extremely dangerous in overdose.

Anticonvulsants: Anticonvulsants used in child psychiatry include gabapentin, pregabalin, valproate, carbamazepine, and oxcarbazepine. All of these are sometimes used for severe anxiety, though usually in the context of comorbid conditions such as mood disorders or developmental disorders. It is important to note that some patients have abused gabapentin and pregabalin, and this risk might guide clinical use with some patients and families.

Antipsychotics: Antipsychotics are sometimes used for severe anxiety—usually, but not always, in combination with other medications. However, given the array of potential side effects (such as weight gain), there are usually better options.

Benzodiazepines: Other than exceptionally controlled and rare use for specific phobias, surgical procedures, and severe childhood schizophrenia, the risks of benzodiazepines in children and adolescents far outweigh the benefits. Common problems include interference in memory and learning, sedation, and reduced motor coordination as well as paradoxical agitation. If you do use them, we recommend choosing those with longer half-lives (such as lorazepam as opposed to alprazolam), using low doses, using them only briefly (days not weeks), being aware of the risk for abuse and diversion, and using them in support of a comprehensive plan that, for chronic conditions, includes psychotherapy.

HYPNOTICS

Sleep disorders, like anxiety disorders, are another area where non-pharmacological approaches should take clear precedence. Teach parents about some basic sleep hygiene measures, such as electronics restrictions, regular schedules, later-morning starts for teens, and regular exercise. If these maneuvers are not successful, try a more definitive intervention like cognitive behavioral therapy for insomnia (CBT-I), which has been shown to be effective. It may be appropriate to consider sleep studies, although in young children these can be more challenging due to discomfort and sorting out issues of separation at night.

Sleep medications should probably be universally restricted in infants and young children due to safety concerns including dependence, delirium, and in some cases death, the latter possibly by inadvertent overdose. The possible exception might be in cases of severe developmental challenges accompanied by persistent and truly intractable insomnia, or perhaps in rare instances of classic early childhood mania.

Some clinicians might try herbal remedies first. Chamomile tea, while mild, is a good first-line off-the-shelf product that goes well with the implementation of better sleep hygiene practices. Valerian, also mild, comes in capsules and is also often helpful, although it sometimes carries an unpleasant odor. While kava is sometimes listed as another "natural herbal" sleep remedy, many people have severe side effects, including intense dreams, over-sedation, intoxication, and physiological dependence. Rare cases of hepatic failure have been reported and are likely due to contaminants, not kava itself.

Our order of medications is roughly the following:

Central alpha agonists and antagonists: Guanfacine and clonidine are often helpful for initiating sleep. Clonidine may last only a few hours and result in rebound insomnia. Prazosin, an alpha antagonist, may help as well, especially in the setting of PTSD with nightmares.

Melatonin: Melatonin, an endogenous sleep hormone, has come into regular use in kids despite mixed studies showing little efficacy and some showing rebound insomnia when discontinued. Early concerns about safety (eg, reports of seizures) have not borne out, and so this medication is mostly seen as benign. Melatonin has a short half-life and may also cause rebound waking at night, although long-acting preparations are now available. Some people report vivid dreaming when they use melatonin.

Ramelteon: This potent melatonin receptor agonist typically requires several weeks to see benefits. Since teens often do not have patience for such a trial, it can be a tough sell for them. Its use in children is relatively rare as most opt for melatonin instead. Still, it is among the more benign sleep medications.

Antihistamines: Diphenhydramine, doxylamine, cyproheptadine, and hydroxyzine are commonly used in both adults and children to induce sleep. All of these may cause delirium or disinhibition. They may be habit-forming and therefore should be used with care. Occasional reports of overdose deaths have also been reported. Recent questions about lifetime cumulative use of anticholinergic medications in adults with later risk for dementia may beg caution in use of diphenhydramine, particularly if there is a known increased lifetime risk of dementia (eg, in Down syndrome or with family history of dementia).

Sedating antidepressants: These medications, including mirtazapine and imipramine, can be useful for helping children and adolescents to sleep. Both mirtazapine and imipramine may create daytime sedation. Mirtazapine contributes more to increase in appetite, and imipramine has more potential for cardiac arrhythmias (particularly in overdose). ECGs should be considered if there is any suspicion of cardiac risk or if dosages exceed any but the smallest available pills. Trazodone, another older antidepressant, is often used in adults with insomnia, although it is prone to cause more daytime cognitive clouding and carries a small risk of priapism. While it is sometimes used in children and adolescents as well, we tend to avoid it due to concerns about cognitive clouding and possible interference in school function, sports, driving, and other activities requiring coordination and clear thinking.

Benzodiazepine hypnotics: We try to avoid benzodiazepines such as temazepam due to risks of rapid dependence and impairment of memory, motor function, and association with falls and motor vehicle accidents. However, benzos may be useful specifically for night terrors or intractable insomnia. In such cases, we recommend a medium half-life medication such as lorazepam to avoid rebound insomnia or morning grogginess, prescribed in a short course as part of a comprehensive intervention plan.

Non-benzodiazepine hypnotics: We also avoid zolpidem, zaleplon, and eszopiclone, partly for the failure of controlled studies of the z-drugs, as well as for the propensity of these medications for eliciting parasomnolent activity. The incidence of sleepwalking, sleep-talking, and other behaviors is higher in children than adults and can include dangerous wandering. Our own direct knowledge of catastrophic events—adult patients driving, cooking, unremembered deals on overnight flights, and in one case a completed suicide—leave us unlikely to prescribe them to children and adolescents despite their popularity and heavy marketing.

TABLE 6: Anxiolytics and Hypnotics

Generic Name (Brand Name) Year FDA Approved [G] denotes generic availability	Relevant FDA Indication(s) (Pediatric indications in bold)	Available Strengths (mg)	Onset of Action (oral)[2]	Half-Life (hours)	Duration of Action (hours)	Usual Pediatric Dosage Range (starting–max) (mg)	Comments
Alprazolam [G] (Xanax, Xanax XR, Niravam) 1981	GAD Panic disorder	Tablets: 0.25, 0.5, 1, 2 ER tablets: 0.5, 1, 2, 3 ODT: 0.25, 0.5, 1, 2 Liquid: 1 mg/mL	30 min (IR, ODT) 1–2 hrs (XR)	11–16	3–4 (IR) 10 (XR)	0.375–3.5 mg/day divided TID	NOT RECOMMENDED. Very limited data showing no benefit over placebo in GAD or school refusal/separation anxiety.
Buspirone [G] (BuSpar[1]) 1986	GAD	Tablets: 5, 7.5, 10, 15, 30	1–2 weeks+	2–3	N/A	5 mg TID–20 mg TID	Very limited data, showing no benefit over placebo in GAD
Clomipramine [G] (Anafranil) 1989	**OCD (10+ yrs)**	25, 50, 75	1–2 weeks+	32	N/A	25 mg QHS–200 mg QHS	Use for OCD if SSRI fails or not tolerated
Clonazepam [G] (Klonopin, Klonopin Wafers[1]) 1975	**Absence, petit mal, akinetic and myoclonic seizures (myoclonia) (≤10 yrs)** Panic disorder; insomnia (off label)	Tablets: 0.5, 1, 2 ODT: 0.125, 0.25, 0.5, 1, 2	1 hr	20–80	4–8	0.125 mg BID–1 mg BID	NOT RECOMMENDED. Very limited data, showing no benefit over placebo in GAD or social phobia.
Clonidine [G] (Catapres) 1976	**ER (Kapvay) approved for ADHD (6–17 yrs)**; anxiety (off label)	IR 0.1, 0.2, 0.3 ER 0.1, 0.2	1 hr	12–16	4–6	0.05–0.4	Used especially when comorbid ADHD or tics; do not stop an ongoing dosage abruptly (rebound hypertension)
Diazepam [G] (Valium, Diastat) 1963	**Seizures and spasm (infants+, but neonate off-label); GAD; alcohol withdrawal; anxiety (short-term) (0.5+ yrs)**	Tablets: 2, 5, 10 Liquid: 5 mg/5 mL, 5 mg/mL Injection: 5 mg/mL Rectal gel: 2.5, 5, 7.5, 10, 12.5, 15, 17.5, 20	30 min	>100	4–6	0.04–0.2 mg/kg Q2–4h PRN (0.5–12 yrs) 2–10 mg BID–QID (≥13 yrs)	NOT RECOMMENDED for anxiety or insomnia. Typically used as one-time dose in emergency, dental, or seizure settings.
Diphenhydramine [G] (Benadryl, others) 1946 Available OTC and Rx	**Insomnia (12+ yrs); Allergy (20+ lbs); motion sickness (6+ yrs)**	Capsule: 25, 50 Liquid: 12.5 mg/mL	1 hr	3.5–9	4–6	6.25–50 QHS	Some benefit in pediatric patients; caution: paradoxical reaction
Doxylamine [G] (Unisom, others) 1978 Available OTC and Rx	**Nighttime sleep aid (12+ yrs); rhinitis (2+ yrs)**	Tablet: 25	1 hr	10	4–6	6.25–50 QHS	Some benefit in pediatric patients; caution: paradoxical reaction
Eszopiclone [G] (Lunesta) 2004	Insomnia (sleep onset and sleep maintenance)	Tablet: 1, 2, 3	30 min	6	6–8	1–3 QHS	NOT RECOMMENDED. No benefit in pediatric patients.
Gabapentin [G] (Neurontin) 1993	Anxiety **Seizures (3+ yrs)**	Capsule: 100, 300, 400 Tablet: 600, 800 Oral solution: 50 mg/mL ER tablet: 300, 600	1–2 hrs	5–7	6–8	100 QHS–300 TID	

Generic Name (Brand Name) Year FDA Approved [G] denotes generic availability	Relevant FDA Indication(s) (Pediatric indications in bold)	Available Strengths (mg)	Onset of Action (oral)[2]	Half-Life (hours)	Duration of Action (hours)	Usual Pediatric Dosage Range (starting–max) (mg)	Comments
Guanfacine IR [G] (Tenex) 1986	ADHD (only ER-approved)	1, 2	1 hr	13–14	N/A	0.5–4 QD (do not increase faster than 1 mg/wk)	Very limited data suggesting improvement in generalized, separation or social anxiety disorder; do not stop abruptly (rebound hypertension); not a 1:1 conversion from IR; do not give with high-fat meals; use especially when comorbid ADHD
Guanfacine ER [G] (Intuniv) 2009	**ADHD (6–17 yrs)**	1, 2, 3, 4	1–2 hrs	13–14	N/A	1–4 QD (do not increase faster than 1 mg/wk) (adolescents 7 mg/day max)	
Hydroxyzine [G] (Atarax, Vistaril) 1956	**Anxiety (6+ yrs); pruritis (<6 yrs by weight)**	Capsule: 25, 50, 100 Tablet: 10, 25, 50 Liquid: 10 mg/5 mL	1 hr	20–25	4–6	12.5–100 QHS	
Imipramine [G] Tofranil brand discontinued; generic only 1984	MDD; **nocturnal enuresis (6+ yrs)**	10, 25, 50, 75, 100, 125, 150	1–2 weeks+	11–25	N/A	10–100 QHS	
Lorazepam [G] (Ativan) 1977	GAD; insomnia (off-label); **anxiety (short-term) (12+ yrs)**	Tablets: 0.5, 1, 2 Liquid: 2 mg/mL Injection: 2 mg/mL, 4 mg/mL	30–60 min	10–20	4–6	0.05 mg/kg Q4–8h PRN; max 2 mg/dose	NOT RECOMMENDED. No benefit in pediatric patients.
Mirtazapine [G] (Remeron) 1996	MDD	Tablet: 7.5, 15, 30, 45; ODT: 15, 30, 45	1–2 weeks+	20–40	N/A	7.5–45 QHS	
Prazosin [G] (Minipress) 1976	PTSD (off-label)	Capsules: 1, 2, 5	1–2 hrs	2–3	4–6	1 mg/day–10 mg/day QHS or divided BID	
Propranolol [G] (Inderal) 1973	Performance anxiety, tremor (off-label)	Tablets: 10, 20, 40, 60, 80	60 min	3–6	4–6	<35 kg: 10–20 mg TID ≥35 kg: 20–40 mg TID	
Temazepam [G] (Restoril) 1981	Insomnia (short-term)	Capsule: 7.5, 15, 22.5, 30	30–60 min	9–18	4–6	7.5–30 QHS	NOT RECOMMENDED. No benefit in pediatric patients.
Trazodone [G] (Desyrel[3], Oleptro[3]) 1981/2010	Depression Insomnia (off-label)	Tablet: 50, 100, 150, 300 ER tablet: 150, 300	1 hr	7–10	Unknown	25–200 QHS	Used especially in kids with depression or anxiety
Triazolam [G] (Halcion) 1982	Insomnia (short-term)	Tablet: 0.125, 0.25	15–30 min	1.5–5.5	Unknown	0.125–0.5 QHS	NOT RECOMMENDED. No benefit in pediatric patients.
Zaleplon [G] (Sonata) 1999	Insomnia (short-term, sleep onset)	Capsule: 5, 10	30 min	1	4	10–20 QHS	NOT RECOMMENDED. No benefit in pediatric patients.

Generic Name (Brand Name) Year FDA Approved [G] denotes generic availability	Relevant FDA Indication(s) (Pediatric indications in bold)	Available Strengths (mg)	Onset of Action (oral)[2]	Half-Life (hours)	Duration of Action (hours)	Usual Pediatric Dosage Range (starting–max) (mg)	Comments
Zolpidem [G] (Ambien, Ambien CR, Edluar, Zolpimist) 1992 Generic not available for Zolpimist or Edluar SL	Insomnia (IR: short-term, sleep onset; CR: sleep onset and maintenance	Tablet: 5, 10 ER tablet: 6.25, 12.5 SL tablet: 5, 10 Oral spray: 5 mg/spray	30 min	2.5–3	6–8	10, 12.5 CR (5, 6.25 in women)	NOT RECOMMENDED. No benefit in pediatric patients.
Zolpidem low dose (Intermezzo) [G] 2011	Difficulty falling asleep after middle-of-the-night awakening	SL tablet: 1.75, 3.5	30 min	2.5	4	1.75 women; 3.5 men	NOT RECOMMENDED. No benefit in pediatric patients.

[1] For approximate benzodiazepine dose equivalencies, refer to Table 8.1
[2] Onset and duration vary from person to person, dose to dose, and preparation to preparation
[3] Brand discontinued; available as generic only

TABLE 6.1: Benzodiazepine Dosage Equivalencies

As noted in the preceding pages, benzodiazepines are generally not recommended for kids. When used, we generally stick to lorazepam or clonazepam. We provide here a table of equivalencies for those cases where you may need to switch a child over to another benzodiazepine.

Benzodiazepine	Approximate Equivalent Dosage (mg)
Alprazolam (Xanax)	0.5
Chlordiazepoxide (Librium)	25
Clonazepam (Klonopin)	0.25–0.5
Clorazepate (Tranxene)	7.5
Diazepam (Valium)	5
Estazolam (ProSom)	1
Flurazepam (Dalmane)	15
Lorazepam (Ativan)	1
Oxazepam (Serax)	15
Quazepam (Doral)	15
Temazepam (Restoril)	15
Triazolam (Halcion)	0.25

ANTIHISTAMINES (Diphenhydramine, Doxylamine, Hydroxyzine) Fact Sheet [G]

PEDIATRIC FDA INDICATIONS:
- Diphenhydramine: **Insomnia** (12–17 years); allergies (20+ lbs); motion sickness (6+ years).
- Doxylamine: **Insomnia** (12+ years); rhinitis (12+ years).
- Hydroxyzine: **Anxiety** (6–17 years); pruritis (<6 years by weight).

ADULT FDA INDICATIONS:
Insomnia; allergies; motion sickness; antiparkinsonism.

OFF-LABEL USES:
EPS; nausea and vomiting (morning sickness).

DOSAGE FORMS:
- Diphenhydramine (G): tablets, chewable tablets, caplets, capsules, and oral solutions, varies by brand: 25 mg, 50 mg. Available as Benadryl, Compoz, Nytol, Simply Sleep, Sleep-Eze, Sominex, Unisom SleepGels, Unisom SleepMelts, and generic.
- Doxylamine (G): tablets: 25 mg. Available as NyQuil, Unisom SleepTabs, and generic.
- Hydroxyzine (G): capsules: 25, 50, 100 mg; tablets: 10, 25, 50 mg; liquid: 10 mg/5 mL; injectable: 25 mg/mL, 50 mg/mL. Available as Atarax, Vistaril, and generic.

PEDIATRIC DOSAGE GUIDANCE:
- Diphenhydramine: Start 25 mg (use 12.5 mg in kids 6–11 years, or 6.25 mg if 2–5 years) 30 minutes before bedtime. The dose required to induce sleep can be as low as 6.25 mg, but usual dose is 25 mg. Some older kids may require 50 mg at bedtime.
- Doxylamine: for insomnia in children 12+ years: 25 mg given 30 minutes before bedtime;
- Hydroxyzine: for children <6 years: 50 mg/day divided or 2 mg/kg/day divided every 6–8 hours, or 15 mg/m2/day given in divided doses; for children ≥6 years: 50–100 mg/day divided, or 2 mg/kg/day divided every 6–8 hours.

MONITORING: No specific monitoring of note.

COST: $

SIDE EFFECTS:
- Most common: dry mouth, ataxia, urinary retention, constipation, drowsiness, memory problems.
- Serious but rare: blurred vision, tachycardia.

MECHANISM, PHARMACOKINETICS, AND DRUG INTERACTIONS:
- Histamine H1 antagonist.
- Metabolized by liver, primarily CYP2D6; t ½: for diphenhydramine, 3.5–9 hours; for doxylamine, 10 hours (12–15 hours in elderly); for hydroxyzine, 20–25 hours.
- Avoid use with other antihistamines or anticholinergics (additive effects).

EVIDENCE AND CLINICAL PEARLS:
- Controlled studies of diphenhydramine and placebo have reported mixed results. Two found it no better than placebo for sleep quality and maintenance in infants, children, and adolescents, while the third found improvement in sleep initiation and maintenance compared to placebo. One study in babies 6–15 months found diphenhydramine no better than placebo.
- These antihistamines non-selectively antagonize central and peripheral histamine H1 receptors. They also have secondary anticholinergic effects, which can cause side effects including dry mouth and urinary retention, as well as cognitive impairment in susceptible populations. Some kids may experience a paradoxical excitation.
- Tolerance may develop over time, necessitating use of higher doses. Best used as short-term sleep aid.
- Be aware that anticholinergic drugs are often used to treat or prevent extrapyramidal symptoms in patients taking antipsychotics; diphenhydramine is often chosen and dosed at night to take advantage of its sedative effect.

FUN FACTS:
The name NyQuil is a portmanteau of "night" and "tranquil."

BOTTOM LINE:
Antihistamines can be effective sleepers for some kids and are the most prescribed by pediatricians, although some patients may experience too much grogginess ("hangover") in the morning or a paradoxical excitation. Good option to keep in your bag of tricks due to low risk of drug tolerance, dependence, or abuse, and experience in kids.

BUSPIRONE (BuSpar) Fact Sheet [G]

PEDIATRIC FDA INDICATIONS:
None.

ADULT FDA INDICATIONS:
Generalized anxiety disorder (GAD).

OFF-LABEL USES:
Treatment-resistant depression; anxiety symptoms in depression.

DOSAGE FORMS:
Tablets (G): 5 mg, 7.5 mg, 10 mg, 15 mg, 30 mg (scored).

PEDIATRIC DOSAGE GUIDANCE:
- No guidance on dosing in children and adolescents.
- Adult dosing: Start 7.5 mg BID or 5 mg TID; increase by increments of 5 mg/day every 2–3 days to target dose 20 mg–30 mg/day divided BID-TID; max 20 mg TID.

MONITORING: No specific monitoring of note.

COST: $

SIDE EFFECTS:
- Most common: dizziness, nervousness, nausea, headache, jitteriness.

MECHANISM, PHARMACOKINETICS, AND DRUG INTERACTIONS:
- Serotonin 5HT1A receptor partial agonist.
- Metabolized primarily through CYP3A4; t ½: 2–3 hours.
- Avoid use with MAOIs; caution with serotonergic agents due to additive effects and risk for serotonin syndrome. Caution with 3A4 inhibitors or inducers as they may affect buspirone serum levels; adjust dose.

EVIDENCE AND CLINICAL PEARLS:
- Although very well-tolerated, randomized placebo-controlled data found buspirone 15–60 mg/day to be no better than placebo in kids 6–17 years with GAD.
- Similar to antidepressants, buspirone requires 1–2 weeks for onset of therapeutic effects, with full effects occurring over several weeks, and offers no "as-needed" benefits.
- Non-sedating, non-habit-forming alternative to benzodiazepines for anxiety, but minimal efficacy data in kids show it may be no better than placebo.

FUN FACT:
Other psychotropic agents with 5HT1A partial agonist effects include aripiprazole, ziprasidone, and vilazodone.

BOTTOM LINE:
Despite the lack of large randomized controlled data to support first-line use, buspirone may be used adjunctively in kids who exhibit partial response to first-line therapies for anxiety (SSRI, SNRI), without the sedation and abuse potential burden of benzodiazepines.

CLONAZEPAM (Klonopin) Fact Sheet [G]

PEDIATRIC FDA INDICATIONS:
Seizure disorders.

ADULT FDA INDICATIONS:
Seizure disorders; panic disorder.

OFF-LABEL USES:
Other anxiety disorders; insomnia; acute mania or psychosis; catatonia.

DOSAGE FORMS:
- **Tablets (G):** 0.5 mg, 1 mg, 2 mg.
- **Orally disintegrating tablets (G):** 0.125 mg, 0.25 mg, 0.5 mg, 1 mg, 2 mg.

PEDIATRIC DOSAGE GUIDANCE:
- Minimal guidance on dosing in children and adolescents.
- Start 0.125 mg–0.25 mg daily, increase by 0.125 mg–0.25 mg/day increments as needed to response; max dose 2 mg/day.
- Dose varies based on patient characteristics (eg, age) and tolerance to benzodiazepines.

MONITORING: No specific monitoring of note.

COST: $

SIDE EFFECTS:
- Most common: somnolence, daytime grogginess, confusion, ataxia.
- Serious but rare: anterograde amnesia, increased fall risk, paradoxical reaction (irritability, agitation); respiratory depression (avoid in patients with sleep apnea).

MECHANISM, PHARMACOKINETICS, AND DRUG INTERACTIONS:
- Binds to benzodiazepine receptors to enhance GABA effects.
- Metabolized primarily through CYP3A4; t ½: 20–80 hours.
- Avoid concomitant use with other CNS depressants, including alcohol and opioids (additive effects). Potent CYP3A4 inhibitors (eg, fluvoxamine, erythromycin) may increase clonazepam levels; CYP3A4 inducers (eg, carbamazepine) may decrease clonazepam levels.

EVIDENCE AND CLINICAL PEARLS:
- Double-blind placebo-controlled data found no benefit over placebo in 15 kids (7–13 years) with GAD or social phobia. Common side effects included irritability, drowsiness, and oppositional behavior.
- C-IV controlled substance.
- High potency, long-acting benzodiazepine with active metabolites that may accumulate.
- Withdrawal effects may not be seen until 3–5 days after abrupt discontinuation and may last 10–14 days due to long half-life and active metabolites of clonazepam.
- Full effects of a particular dose may not be evident for a few days since active metabolites will accumulate with continual use (versus PRN use). Wait several days before increasing dose if patient is taking clonazepam regularly.

FUN FACT:
Klonopin tablets (or "K-pins") have a street value of $2–$5 per tablet, depending on dose and geographic region.

BOTTOM LINE:
Despite the lack of large randomized controlled data to support its use, clonazepam may be used, very short-term, adjunctively in kids who exhibit only partial response to first-line therapies (SSRI, SNRI) or have severe anxiety.

LORAZEPAM (Ativan) Fact Sheet [G]

PEDIATRIC FDA INDICATIONS:
None.

ADULT FDA INDICATIONS:
Generalized anxiety disorder (GAD); status epilepticus (IV route).

OFF-LABEL USES:
Other anxiety disorders; insomnia; acute mania or psychosis; catatonia; preoperative sedation; chemo-related nausea/vomiting.

DOSAGE FORMS:
- **Tablets (G):** 0.5 mg, 1 mg, 2 mg.
- **Oral concentrate (G):** 2 mg/mL.
- **Injection (G):** 2 mg/mL, 4 mg/mL.

PEDIATRIC DOSAGE GUIDANCE:
- Anxiety: 0.05 mg/kg Q4–8h PRN; max 2 mg/dose.
- Insomnia (off-label use): Start 0.25 mg–1 mg QHS, 20–30 minutes before bedtime; max 2 mg nightly.

MONITORING: No specific monitoring of note.

COST: $

SIDE EFFECTS:
- Most common: somnolence, dizziness, weakness, ataxia.
- Serious but rare: anterograde amnesia, increased fall risk, paradoxical reaction (irritability, agitation); respiratory depression (avoid in patients with sleep apnea).

MECHANISM, PHARMACOKINETICS, AND DRUG INTERACTIONS:
- Binds to benzodiazepine receptors to enhance GABA effects.
- Metabolism primarily hepatic (non-CYP450) to inactive compounds; t ½: 10–20 hours.
- Avoid concomitant use with other CNS depressants, including alcohol and opioids (additive effects). No risk for CYP450 drug interactions.

EVIDENCE AND CLINICAL PEARLS:
- There are no pediatric studies in anxiety disorders. Evidence is mainly for pre-procedure single-dose use.
- C-IV controlled substance.
- Lorazepam does not have a long half-life or active metabolites that could accumulate, and it poses no CYP450 drug interaction risk.
- Withdrawal symptoms are usually seen on the first day after abrupt discontinuation and last 5–7 days in patients receiving short-intermediate half-life benzodiazepines such as lorazepam. A gradual taper is highly recommended, particularly if prolonged treatment on a high dose.
- Tolerance to sedative effect may develop within 2–4 weeks of use, and benzodiazepines affect the normal sleep architecture; thus, long-term use is discouraged.

FUN FACT:
Early Ativan marketing efforts included clever direct-to-consumer advertising campaigns. These included: "Now it can be yours—The Ativan experience" in 1977 and "In a world where certainties are few … no wonder Ativan is prescribed by so many caring clinicians" in 1987.

BOTTOM LINE:
Benzodiazepines are generally only appropriate for use before procedures. Lorazepam probably has less risk of abuse than others.

PRAZOSIN (Minipress) Fact Sheet [G]

PEDIATRIC FDA INDICATIONS:
None.

ADULT FDA INDICATIONS:
Hypertension.

OFF-LABEL USES:
PTSD.

DOSAGE FORMS:
Capsules (G): 1 mg, 2 mg, 5 mg.

PEDIATRIC DOSAGE GUIDANCE:
- PTSD (off-label): Doses studied are 0.02–0.3 mg/kg given at bedtime; titrate dose slowly to minimize possibility of "first-dose" orthostatic hypotension. Start 1 mg QHS x 3 days, increase slowly based on response. Target 1 mg–5 mg/day; doses up to 15 mg daily studied.
- May dose-divide BID to target daytime PTSD-associated arousal symptoms.

MONITORING: BP.

COST: $

SIDE EFFECTS:
- Most common: somnolence, dizziness, headache, weakness.
- Serious but rare: orthostasis and syncope; prolonged erections and priapism have been reported.

MECHANISM, PHARMACOKINETICS, AND DRUG INTERACTIONS:
- Alpha-1 adrenergic receptor antagonist.
- Metabolism primarily hepatic (non-CYP450); t ½: 2–3 hours.
- Caution with other antihypertensive agents, diuretics, and PDE5 inhibitors (eg, Viagra) that may have additive hypotensive effects.

EVIDENCE AND CLINICAL PEARLS:
- Initial studies in adults showed improvement in trauma-related nightmares and sleep quality when dosed at bedtime. Subsequent randomized controlled trials have shown positive effects on daytime PTSD symptoms also when dosed BID.
- A retrospective chart review of 34 kids (5–18 years) with PTSD suggested prazosin is well-tolerated and associated with improvements in nightmares and sleep.

FUN FACT:
Prazosin is an effective drug for kids in the treatment of serious scorpion envenomations with significant sympathetic symptoms.

BOTTOM LINE:
Although there are only minimal data, consider prazosin for PTSD in kids, especially for PTSD-associated sleep disturbances and nightmares, but monitor BP.

PROPRANOLOL (Inderal) Fact Sheet [G]

PEDIATRIC FDA INDICATIONS:
None.

ADULT FDA INDICATIONS:
Hypertension; angina; post-MI cardioprotection; atrial fibrillation; migraine prophylaxis; essential tremor.

OFF-LABEL USES:
Performance anxiety; tremor due to medication side effects (especially lithium).

DOSAGE FORMS:
Tablets (G): 10 mg, 20 mg, 40 mg, 60 mg, 80 mg (scored).

PEDIATRIC DOSAGE GUIDANCE:
- Minimal guidance on dosing in children and adolescents.
- Start 5 mg–10 mg QD, increase by 5 mg/day increments as needed to response; max dose 20 mg/day. May divide dose BID.
- Performance anxiety (off-label use): Give 10 mg about 60 minutes prior to performance; usual effective dose for most is 10 mg–20 mg.
- Medication-induced tremor: Start 10 mg BID as needed, can go up to 30 mg–120 mg daily in two or three divided doses. Can also use Inderal LA, long-acting version of propranolol, 60 mg–80 mg once a day.

MONITORING: BP/P.

COST: $

SIDE EFFECTS:
- Most common: dizziness, fatigue, bradycardia, and hypotension.
- Theoretically may exacerbate asthma symptoms, although studies are equivocal.

MECHANISM, PHARMACOKINETICS, AND DRUG INTERACTIONS:
- Non-selective beta-1 and beta-2 adrenergic receptor antagonist.
- Metabolized primarily through CYP2D6, also 1A2 and 2C19; t ½: 3–6 hours. Be careful about inadvertent increase with fluoxetine leading to fatigue that might be misinterpreted as increased depression.
- Caution with other antihypertensives (additive effects). CYP2D6 inhibitors, and inhibitors or inducers of 1A2 and 2C19, may affect propranolol levels.

EVIDENCE AND CLINICAL PEARLS:
- No data for treating anxiety in children.
- With beta blockade, propranolol reduces some of the somatic symptoms of anxiety (tremor, sweating, flushing, tachycardia).

FUN FACT:
The list of notable people who suffer or have suffered from performance anxiety or stage fright is long. It includes Barbra Streisand, Carly Simon, Van Morrison, Frédéric Chopin, Renée Fleming, Jay Mohr, Hugh Grant, Laurence Olivier, Mahatma Gandhi, and Thomas Jefferson, among others.

BOTTOM LINE:
May be effective and safe for use in performance anxiety, particularly when the sedating or cognitive side effects of benzos could interfere with an individual's performance, but there are no data in kids.

Complementary Treatments

Complementary treatments are popular among patients and their parents, but they are a mixed bag: Some are useful and safe, while others can be hazardous. Contrary to common assumptions, "natural" doesn't equal safe. With this in mind, it is important to always ask patients and families about all the products that they are using. The fact sheets in this section detail potential uses of some of these agents in child psychiatry. Few of these treatments are FDA-approved for use in adults, and none are FDA-approved for use in children. Clinicians need to use their best judgment and ensure that there is clear informed consent covering potential risks, benefits, and unknowns when talking with patients and families about these treatments.

If you are interested in complementary treatments (also known as natural and alternative medicine, or CAM), you will likely recommend various strategies other than the products we cover in this section. These would include exercise (helpful for depression and for preventing cognitive impairment), light therapy (for seasonal affective disorder), massage, meditation, and other modalities. CAM is often used alongside ongoing medication treatment, or it can be used alone. Be careful to consider interactions, such as use of multiple serotonergic agents.

We have included fact sheets on those natural products that have been shown to be effective via standard randomized controlled trials. Some natural products not included here might be effective but have not been adequately tested vs placebo.

Because most of these products are not regulated by the FDA, there are quality control issues. The amounts of active constituents can vary not only from brand to brand, but also from batch to batch, and some products may be adulterated with other herbs, chemicals, drugs, or toxins. Some people feel "pharmaceutical grade" (99% pure) products are better. We recommend that patients stick to well-known brands sold by trusted retailers, ideally with a label that specifies certification by organizations such as U. S. Pharmacopeia (USP), NSF International, or ConsumerLab.com. Seals of approval from these organizations don't guarantee therapeutic efficacy or safety, but although not every batch is tested, the seals indicate that the product contains the amount of the ingredient listed on the label and isn't contaminated with toxins or bacteria. Manufacturers must pay for the testing and certification; hence only a small fraction of supplements carry these seals.

For additional information, you may also find these resources helpful:

- NIH National Center for Complementary and Integrative Health: https://nccih.nih.gov/health/herbsataglance.htm
- National Library of Medicine: https://medlineplus.gov/druginfo/herb_All.html
- Natural Medicines Comprehensive Database (requires subscription): http://naturaldatabase.therapeuticresearch.com
- Consumer Lab (requires subscription): http://www.consumerlab.com

COMMONLY USED COMPLEMENTARY TREATMENTS

The complementary treatments that clinicians may recommend most frequently are omega-3 fatty acids for people on antipsychotics, melatonin for sleep, and L-methylfolate for people with either proven or suspected methylenetetrahydrofolate reductase (MTHFR) deficiency.

Omega-3 fatty acids: Omega-3s have some limited research that suggests they may reduce relapse risk in bipolar disorder, may be beneficial in depression or ADHD, and may reduce the risk of tardive dyskinesia in children and adolescents who are on antipsychotics. A recent AHRQ comparative effectiveness review of a number of studies concluded that omega-3 supplementation as monotherapy or as augmentation was ineffective for ADHD in kids.

Melatonin: Melatonin is often helpful for sleep but can cause rebound wakefulness during the night, create vivid dreams, and rebound insomnia when discontinued. Early reports of seizures have not been borne out, nor have concerns about melatonin causing hormonal problems. As always, use the minimum effective dose, usually 0.3–3 mg in children, perhaps up to 5 mg.

L-methylfolate: Another relatively recent newcomer, L-methylfolate has been medicalized by the marketing of a prescription form and the growing popularity of MTHFR genetic testing. Because the evidence base for this practice is growing, we often test for MTHFR, particularly in depressed children and teens who are not responding to antidepressant treatment. Occasionally there are clear results showing enzymatic deficiency, and apparent improvement with supplementation.

LESS COMMON BUT NOTABLE TREATMENTS

N-acetylcysteine (NAC): An amino acid, NAC may help anxiety, skin picking, and obsessive-compulsive symptoms with no ill effects.

Ginkgo biloba: Ginkgo biloba is potentially helpful for symptoms of ADHD. We will often use it as a way to ease an understandably cautious family into more effective treatment, such as a stimulant. Ginkgo is generally considered to be safe;

however, there are reports of a low but notable risk of stroke, which may have relevance for children or adolescents with medical conditions.

S-adenosyl-L-methionine (SAMe) and St. John's wort: SAMe and St. John's wort are widely touted to help mild to moderate depression in adults, presumably via serotonergic mechanisms similar to SSRIs. St. John's wort is routinely used in Europe. However, as with most supplements available in the US, the dosage is variable due to poor oversight of the industry and high pill-to-pill variability. We recommend caution in children due to risks of hyperserotonergic syndromes, particularly in combination with SSRIs or SNRIs, and perhaps triptan medications used for migraine.

Low-dose naltrexone (LDN): LDN is becoming popular as well. Doses typically used are on the order of 0.06 mg/kg/day, or about 2–4 mg/day in most kids. Since naltrexone is only available in 50 mg tablets, families are relying on compounding pharmacies to prepare these ultra-low doses. LDN may be helpful for anxiety and agitation, particularly in people with autism spectrum disorder (ASD). It has also been used for fibromyalgia, fatigue, and dissociation. While liver function testing is recommended when prescribing naltrexone for substance use treatment (usual dose 25–50 mg daily), the risks of LDN are probably minimal. Efficacy data to support these uses are minimal, at best.

Oxytocin: Oxytocin is enjoying wider popularity as well, currently in the form of a nasal spray used twice a day at doses of 10–40 micrograms per dose. Research is mixed for improved social function in adults with ASD and negligible for children. There is a theoretical concern that oxytocin might lead a vulnerable child to attach to any stranger; however, this has not borne out.

Vitamin D: Reports of population-wide vitamin D deficiency and its possible association with depression and other health conditions are fueling a surge of supplementation. Vitamin D levels (25-OH vitamin D) seem to be the lab test du jour. Should we all be testing for vitamin D in children and teens? Perhaps, especially since we typically advise parents to be sure children are using sunscreen—its use lowers the risk for melanoma but also limits the natural production of vitamin D. Note that there are potential dangers in over-supplementation (greater than 5000 IU per day of vitamin D3 in adults), which can create osteoporosis secondary to hypercalcemia, renal toxicity, and hepatotoxicity.

Vitamin A supplementation: Often among the mega-vitamin treatments touted for children with developmental and learning challenges, vitamin A is also toxic in high doses: 2000 IU (600 mcg) for infants and young children ages 0–3, 3000 IU (900 mcg) for ages 4–8, 5667 IU (1700 mcg) for ages 9–13, and 9333 IU (2300 mcg) for ages 14–18.

Methyl B12 injections for autism: These are among the most common of the "biomedical" treatments in the autism world, and as usual, the research is mixed except for the open-label cases where families report that the injections are helpful. This is probably harmless, though weekly injections can traumatize susceptible children, and injection site complications are possible.

Intravenous immunoglobulin (IVIG): IVIG is also frequently used with children with developmental challenges; in particular, it is thought by some to be helpful for ill-defined immunological dyscrasias associated with ASD. Reports of positive effects in non-controlled settings are, in our view, rendered moot by the risk of giving people pooled blood products. Nevertheless, IVIG is FDA-approved and prescribed in other medical conditions such as primary immunodeficiency syndromes and leukemia, so it may make sense in certain circumstances if a child has such a comorbid condition.

D-cycloserine: Early studies indicated that the amino acid d-cycloserine could boost the effectiveness of cognitive behavioral therapy (CBT) when administered prior to therapy sessions, especially for OCD. More recent negative studies have tempered that enthusiasm.

Magnesium supplementation: While there is some risk associated with overuse of magnesium, there are fairly consistent reports of people who have reduced anxiety when using magnesium supplementation in children, adolescents, and adults.

TREATMENTS THAT ARE NOT RECOMMENDED

Cannabinoids: Cannabinoids (CBD) are a component of marijuana that do not produce a high and are believed by some to help depression and schizophrenia. Safety and efficacy studies, however, are limited to 2 good studies demonstrating efficacy in treating intractable seizures. Tetrahydrocannabinol (THC) doubles psychosis risk and reduces motivation, adding to concerns about CBD. Illegal by federal law, clinicians need to weigh whether to recuse themselves from care or even contact protective services if they learn that a patient is using or being given CBD. Consultation and documentation may be more critical in this scenario.

Several agents purported to be beneficial for psychiatric symptoms but have no evidence to support their use include secretin, colloidal silver, and pycnogenol. We do not recommend their use.

Secretin: Secretin is a gastrointestinal hormone that has been used experimentally for autism. The studies have been negative, and there are significant potential hazards. For example, one secretin infusion-related death was reported a number of years ago.

Colloidal silver: This is sometimes used to treat autism. However, there are no controlled efficacy studies. Side effects include permanent graying of skin.

Pycnogenol: Pycnogenol is an alleged antioxidant extracted from grape seeds and pine tree bark. It has been reportedly used for autism, but no legitimate research has been published, and the cost of the treatment is high.

TABLE 7: Complementary Treatments

Name (Brand Name, if applicable)	Commonly Available Strengths (mg)	Reported Uses in Psychiatry	Usual Pediatric Dosage Range (starting–max) (mg)
L-Methylfolate (Deplin and others)	0.4, 0.8, 1, 3, 5, 7.5, 15	Depression (adjunct)	15
Magnesium	100, 250, 400, 500	Anxiety, ADHD	65–350
Melatonin	0.5, 1, 2.5, 3, 5, 10	Insomnia	0.3–5
N-Acetylcysteine	500, 600, 750, 1000	OCD, trichotillomania, nail biting, skin picking	1200–2400
Omega-3 Fatty Acids (Fish Oil)	500, 1000, 1200	Depression (unipolar, bipolar, and ADHD, albeit evidence not supportive for ADHD)	500–2000
S-Adenosyl-L-Methionine (SAMe)	100, 200, 400	Depression	800 BID
St. John's Wort	100, 300, 450	Depression	300 TID
Vitamin D	1000 IU, 2000 IU, 5000 IU, 10,000 IU (as D3)	Depression	1000–2500 IU

L-METHYLFOLATE (Deplin) Fact Sheet

PEDIATRIC AND ADULT FDA INDICATIONS:
None.

OFF-LABEL USES:
Adjunctive treatment for depression (considered a "medical food product" by the FDA, not an FDA-approved drug product, although available as prescription only).

DOSAGE FORMS:
- **Capsules (Deplin):** 7.5 mg, 15 mg.
- **Tablets and capsules (various other L-methylfolate products):** 0.4 mg, 0.8 mg, 1 mg, 3 mg, 5 mg.

PEDIATRIC DOSAGE GUIDANCE:
- No guidance for pediatric dosing.
- Adult dosing for depression (Deplin only): Start 7.5 mg QD; target and max dose 15 mg/day.

COST: G: $$; Deplin: $$$

SIDE EFFECTS:
- Most common: not well known; likely well-tolerated.
- Serious but rare: Folic acid supplementation may mask symptoms of vitamin B12 deficiency (administration of folic acid may reverse the hematological signs of B12 deficiency, including megaloblastic anemia, while not addressing neurological manifestations). L-methylfolate may be less likely than folic acid to mask B12 deficiency, though the possibility should be considered.

MECHANISM, PHARMACOKINETICS, AND DRUG INTERACTIONS:
- May enhance synthesis of monoamine neurotransmitters.
- No typical drug metabolism pathway as it is naturally stored and used by body; t ½: 3 hours.
- Drug interactions generally unlikely, although L-methylfolate may decrease anticonvulsant levels (including carbamazepine, valproic acid). Drugs that lower folate, such as anticonvulsants (including carbamazepine, valproic acid, lamotrigine), may necessitate higher doses of L-methylfolate.

EVIDENCE AND CLINICAL PEARLS:
- A few small studies in adults over the years have shown that both folate (over the counter) and L-methylfolate may be somewhat helpful as adjunctive agents in the treatment of depression, particularly in those with low baseline folate levels. No studies in pediatric patients.
- Clinicians tend to order genetic testing for MTHFR when a person's symptoms are not improving or a family member has been found to have this problem.
- Dietary folic acid is normally transformed to L-methylfolate by the enzyme MTHFR, and L-methylfolate is necessary for the synthesis of monoamines (serotonin, norepinephrine, dopamine). The marketing pitch for prescribing Deplin is that in about 50% of the population, genetic variations impair the function of MTHFR, leading to low levels of methylfolate. A recent review of the data on one of these genetic polymorphisms (called C677T) found that overall, it did not put people at any higher risk of depression (in fact, schizophrenia was more common).

FUN FACT:
"Medical foods" are foods that are specially formulated and intended for the dietary management of a disease that has distinctive nutritional needs that cannot be met by normal diet alone. These include total parenteral nutrition as well as nasogastric tube feeds and oral rehydration products. Depression has no accepted distinctive nutritional needs.

BOTTOM LINE:
Though the data are not robust, folate supplementation *might* be effective for some kids with depression, but we recommend that patients try the cheap stuff (folic acid) before springing for Deplin (L-methylfolate).

MAGNESIUM Fact Sheet

PEDIATRIC AND ADULT FDA INDICATIONS:
None.

OFF-LABEL USES:
Anxiety; ADHD.

DOSAGE FORMS:
Capsules, tablets, softgels, chewables, oral liquid: 100 mg, 250 mg, 400 mg, 500 mg.

PEDIATRIC DOSAGE GUIDANCE:
- Anxiety: max 65 mg/day for kids 1–3 years; max 110 mg/day for kids 4–8 years; max 350 mg/day for kids >8 years.
- ADHD: Magnesium aspartates and lactates 6 mg/kg/day.

COST: $

SIDE EFFECTS:
- Most common: well-tolerated, although higher doses may cause loose stools and diarrhea.
- Serious but rare: Excessive intake can lead to symptomatic hypermagnesemia, which presents as hypotension, nausea, vomiting, and bradycardia.

MECHANISM, PHARMACOKINETICS, AND DRUG INTERACTIONS:
- Essential mineral used in the human body, as a cofactor.
- Excreted in urine; t ½: unknown.
- Drug interactions generally unlikely.

EVIDENCE AND CLINICAL PEARLS:
- An overview of 18 studies in adults suggested magnesium had a beneficial effect on subjective anxiety; however, they were all poor-quality studies, and the review recommended better controlled trials.
- Magnesium supplements are formulated as various salts (citrate, chloride, gluconate, aspartate, oxide, pidolate, and orotate) or combined with other ingredients (eg, multivitamin).
- Used most often to prevent or treat deficiency or as a laxative. It is sometimes used for pregnancy-induced leg cramps or restless legs syndrome.
- In kids, it may be used for treating anxiety. Magnesium is frequently mentioned in treatment of anxiety in autism; however, research beyond case reports is lacking.
- Although the Natural Medicines database deems magnesium "insufficient reliable evidence to rate," 1 study suggests that elemental magnesium 300 mg/day (adults, mostly women) combined with hawthorn and California poppy (not available in the US) may be useful in the treatment of mild to moderate anxiety.
- Also considered "insufficient reliable evidence to rate" is magnesium's role in children with ADHD. Preliminary data (no randomized, placebo-controlled trials) suggest supplementation may improve hyperactivity in children with ADHD who have low magnesium levels.

FUN FACT:
- In 1618, a farmer in Epsom, England had cows who were refusing to drink from a local well. It turned out the water had a bitter taste but healed scratches and rashes. Thus was the birth of the magnesium compound: epsom salts ($MgSO_4\text{-}7H_2O$).

BOTTOM LINE:
- Magnesium supplementation may improve symptoms of ADHD or anxiety in children with a deficiency, but supporting or convincing evidence is lacking.

MELATONIN Fact Sheet

PEDIATRIC AND ADULT FDA INDICATIONS:
None.

OFF-LABEL USES:
Insomnia; jet lag; work-shift sleep disorder.

DOSAGE FORMS:
Supplied over the counter (OTC) in various forms, including liquid, tablet, capsule, sublingual, and time-release formulations; usually in 0.5 mg, 1 mg, 2.5 mg, 3 mg, 5 mg, and 10 mg.

PEDIATRIC DOSAGE GUIDANCE:
- Doses studied vary from 0.3 mg to 5 mg, and up to 5 mg–10 mg for children with special needs, given 30 minutes–3 hours before bedtime.
- For very young children, use 0.3 mg–1 mg. For school-aged children, use 2.5 mg–5 mg. Some older kids and adolescents, especially those with ASD, may need up to 5 mg–10 mg nightly.
- Insomnia (adults): 0.5 mg–20 mg in early evening. Emerging data suggest lower doses are effective; start low (0.5 mg–1 mg) and gradually increase to desired effect ("normal" melatonin levels vary widely among individuals, and same dose can induce different levels depending on age or health).
- For jet lag, 1 mg–3 mg on day of departure at a time that corresponds to the anticipated bedtime at arrival destination, followed by 1 mg–3 mg at bedtime for next 3–5 days.
- For delayed sleep phase syndrome, 300–500 mcg given 4 hours before bedtime for about 3 weeks, until bedtime is adjusted to desired earlier time.

COST: $

SIDE EFFECTS:
- Most common: generally well-tolerated in the short term. Only rare and mild side effects. Drowsiness, headaches, and dizziness most common but at similar rates to placebo; next-day grogginess or irritability (higher doses); vivid dreams or nightmares (higher doses).
- Serious but rare: No serious side effects reported; however, long-term human studies have not been conducted.

MECHANISM, PHARMACOKINETICS, AND DRUG INTERACTIONS:
- Melatonin receptor agonist.
- Metabolized primarily through CYP1A2, may inhibit CYP1A2; t ½: 35–50 minutes.
- Some suggest melatonin may reduce glucose tolerance and insulin sensitivity and may ↑ efficacy of calcium channel blockers for blood pressure.

EVIDENCE AND CLINICAL PEARLS:
- Melatonin is secreted from the pineal gland in a 24-hour circadian rhythm. It rises at sunset and peaks in the middle of the night, regulating the normal sleep/wake cycle.
- Good evidence and safety database in kids, much of it in kids with ADHD or ASD, and considered a first-line agent in many when pharmacologic intervention is indicated. Studied in kids as young as 3 years.
- A Dutch study followed kids taking melatonin for a mean of 3.1 years and found no significant long-term effects, including pubertal development.

FUN FACT:
Foods containing melatonin include cherries, bananas, grapes, rice, cereals, herbs, olive oil, wine, and beer.

BOTTOM LINE:
Short-term melatonin treatment appears to have only a modest effect size in kids with insomnia. It modestly reduces the time it takes to fall asleep (about 12 minutes) and does not appear to significantly improve overall sleep time. However, some patients and parents report minor improvement in subjective feelings of sleep quality.

N-ACETYLCYSTEINE (NAC) Fact Sheet

PEDIATRIC AND ADULT FDA INDICATIONS:
None.

OFF-LABEL USES:
Obsessive-compulsive disorder (OCD); trichotillomania; nail biting; skin picking.

DOSAGE FORMS:
Capsules: 500 mg, 600 mg, 750 mg, 1000 mg.

PEDIATRIC DOSAGE GUIDANCE:
- Minimal dosing guidance in pediatric patients.
- NAC doses studied have ranged from 600 mg to 6000 mg/day with majority of the studies using 1200–2400 mg/day. Divide dose BID to minimize GI side effects.

COST: $

SIDE EFFECTS:
- Most common: usually well-tolerated with nausea/vomiting, diarrhea, cramping, flatulence being most common side effects. GI symptoms usually diminish after a few weeks.
- Serious but rare: may exacerbate asthma.

MECHANISM, PHARMACOKINETICS, AND DRUG INTERACTIONS:
- NAC is derived from the amino acid cysteine, a precursor of a key brain antioxidant, glutathione. It works as a glutamate modulator, which may have effects on oxidative stress, mitochondrial dysfunction, inflammatory mediators, neurotransmission, and neural plasticity.
- Metabolized extensively by liver with minimal P450 involvement; t ½: 6 hours.
- No known drug interactions; not likely an issue for the majority of patients.

EVIDENCE AND CLINICAL PEARLS:
- Amino acid derivate with antioxidant properties.
- NAC is most recognized for its use as a treatment for acetaminophen overdose.
- Although NAC has been studied in autism, Alzheimer's, cocaine and cannabis addiction, bipolar disorder, depression, trichotillomania, nail biting, skin picking, OCD, and schizophrenia, the results are generally mixed. Best data are in patients with OCD, trichotillomania, nail biting, and skin picking (including Prader-Willi syndrome).
- Majority of data are in adults. Data in kids are limited to case reports and a small (n = 34) randomized clinical trial in kids with OCD, which showed statistically significant improvement in the group that had NAC added to citalopram compared to placebo and citalopram.

FUN FACT:
Many of the published studies have come from an individual Australian researcher who holds a patent on a particular formulation of NAC, raising the issue of bias or a potential conflict of interest.

BOTTOM LINE:
Efficacy of NAC in a wide-ranging number of psychiatric disorders has been investigated. For now, it is best reserved as an add-on for kids only partially responding to SSRIs in OCD or the other repetitive behaviors involving hair, nails, and skin.

OMEGA-3 FATTY ACIDS (Fish Oil) Fact Sheet

PEDIATRIC FDA INDICATIONS:
None.

ADULT FDA INDICATIONS:
High triglycerides (as Lovaza); no FDA indications in psychiatry.

OFF-LABEL USES:
Unipolar and bipolar depression; prevention of tardive dyskinesia; maintenance of mood stability for bipolar disorder.

DOSAGE FORMS:
- Supplied over the counter in various dosages and formulations; 500 mg, 1000 mg, and 1200 mg softgel capsules most common.
- By prescription only: Lovaza: 1000 mg softgel capsules (GSK). Dosage on label usually reflects fish oil dosage, which is not the same as omega-3 fatty acid dosage (eg, 1000 mg fish oil in some brands may provide 300 mg of omega-3 fatty acids, including EPA and DHA). Dosing recommendations are based on mg of fish oil.

PEDIATRIC DOSAGE GUIDANCE:
Effective dose unclear, but studies in children have used 300 mg–1.5 g QD. For depression, start 500 mg/day, increase as tolerated (target dose 1 g–2 g/day); doses >2–3 g/day should be used cautiously. Dividing dose BID–TID helps with side effect tolerability. For ADHD, typical dosages are 1200 mg–1500 mg daily with EPA higher than DHA.

COST: $

SIDE EFFECTS:
- Most common: well-tolerated up to 4 g/day. Nausea, loose stools, fishy aftertaste.
- Serious but rare: Caution in those who are allergic to seafood. Increased risk of bleeding, particularly at higher doses.

MECHANISM, PHARMACOKINETICS, AND DRUG INTERACTIONS:
- Exact mechanism unknown, but may improve cell membrane fluidity and membrane function, change neurotransmitter binding, and promote anti-inflammatory effects.
- Metabolism is hepatic, primarily through CYP450; t ½: unknown.
- For most patients, drug interactions not likely an issue; however, may prolong bleeding time. Fish oils may lower blood pressure and have additive effects when used with antihypertensives.

EVIDENCE AND CLINICAL PEARLS:
- A meta-analysis of 10 trials in 699 children with ADHD treated with omega-3 showed modest efficacy. However, a recent AHRQ Comparative Effectiveness Review concluded omega-3 supplementation is not effective for ADHD based on review of a number of studies of kids with ADHD. While evidence is lacking, omega-3 is used at times for ADHD, and so we have included it here.
- Fish oils contain eicosapentaenoic acid (EPA) and docosahexaenoic acid (DHA); both are omega-3 fatty acids (which form the lipid bilayers of cell membranes). Although the body can synthesize these fats from alpha-linolenic acid (ALA), this is believed to be inefficient in many people.
- Mercury accumulates in fish meat more than in fish oil, which might explain the lack of detectable mercury in most fish oil supplements. Also, questions about increased bleeding risk have not been borne out in research studies.
- Look for formulations with higher EPA than DHA content.
- Omega-3 fatty acids appear helpful as augmentation in unipolar depression in some individual studies, but several meta-analyses have not been able to show robust benefit.

FUN FACT:
Inuit people have been reported to ingest up to 16 g/day (via fish) with no dangerous side effects.

BOTTOM LINE:
Based on the limited data available, the best use of omega-3 fatty acids (particularly 1 g–2 g with at least 60% EPA) is as an adjunct in the treatment of unipolar and bipolar depression.

S-ADENOSYL-L-METHIONINE (SAMe) Fact Sheet

PEDIATRIC AND ADULT FDA INDICATIONS:
None.

OFF-LABEL USES:
Depression; osteoarthritis; cirrhosis and fatty liver disease.

DOSAGE FORMS:
Supplied over the counter most often as 100 mg, 200 mg, 400 mg tablets, usually enteric-coated.

PEDIATRIC DOSAGE GUIDANCE:
- No pediatric dosage guidance.
- Effective dose is variable, but most adult antidepressant studies have used doses of about 400 mg–1600 mg/day (1600 mg most common), usually divided BID.

COST: $

SIDE EFFECTS:
- Most common: well-tolerated. Higher doses may result in flatulence, nausea, vomiting, diarrhea, constipation, dry mouth, headache, mild insomnia, anorexia, sweating, dizziness, and nervousness. Anxiety and tiredness have occurred in people with depression, and hypomania has occurred in people with bipolar disorder.
- Serious but rare: theoretical concern of elevated homocysteine since SAMe is converted to this during normal metabolism. No reports to date, but some recommend taking folate and vitamin B supplements anyway.

MECHANISM, PHARMACOKINETICS, AND DRUG INTERACTIONS:
- Methyl group donor that may increase synthesis of neurotransmitters, increase responsiveness of neurotransmitter receptors, and increase fluidity of cell membranes through the production of phospholipids.
- Metabolism similar to endogenous SAMe (transmethylation, trans-sulphuration, and amino-propylation); t ½: 100 minutes.
- No drug interactions reported. Theoretically, serotonin syndrome possible, but risk is likely minimal.

EVIDENCE AND CLINICAL PEARLS:
- Only 1 small study (n = 3) in pediatric depression showed SAMe 400 mg–1200 mg/day improved symptoms and was well-tolerated.
- SAMe is difficult to formulate as a stable oral salt, and the FDA halted trials of an investigational prescription product in 1993 due to concerns about tablet dissolution; concerns have been raised that some supplements may also have these problems.

FUN FACTS:
SAMe has been available as a dietary supplement in the US since 1999, but it has been used as a prescription drug in Italy since 1979, in Spain since 1985, and in Germany since 1989. Patients in trials of SAMe for depression noted improvement in their arthritis symptoms, suggesting another possible use.

BOTTOM LINE:
Very minimal data in pediatric patients. Consider using it for those patients with mild to moderate depression who are interested in using alternative therapies, or as an augmentation strategy in partial responders.

ST. JOHN'S WORT Fact Sheet

PEDIATRIC AND ADULT FDA INDICATIONS:
None.

OFF-LABEL USES:
Depression.

DOSAGE FORMS:
Supplied over the counter most commonly as 100 mg, 300 mg, 450 mg tablets and capsules.

PEDIATRIC DOSAGE GUIDANCE:
- For mild to moderate depression, most clinical trials have used St. John's wort extract containing 0.3% hypericin and/or 3% hyperforin. Most common dose is 300 mg TID; doses of 1200 mg QD have also been used.
- Some studies have used a 0.2% hypericin extract dosed at 250 mg BID.
- A St. John's wort extract standardized to 5% hyperforin and dosed at 300 mg TID has also been used.

COST: $

SIDE EFFECTS:
- Most common: well-tolerated at recommended doses. Insomnia (decrease dose or take in morning), vivid dreams, restlessness, anxiety, agitation, irritability, gastrointestinal discomfort, diarrhea, fatigue, dry mouth, dizziness, and headache reported. Sexual dysfunction may occur, but less often than with SSRIs.
- Serious but rare: risk of severe phototoxic skin reactions and photosensitivity at high doses (2–4 grams/day).

MECHANISM, PHARMACOKINETICS, AND DRUG INTERACTIONS:
- Thought to exert antidepressant effects by modulating effects of monoamines, and may inhibit reuptake of these neurotransmitters.
- Metabolized primarily through the liver; t ½: 24–48 hours.
- Avoid concomitant use with serotonergic agents: rare cases of serotonin syndrome reported. Potent inducer of many CYP450 enzymes (3A4, 2C9, 1A2) and p-glycoprotein transporter, which results in increased metabolism and reduced plasma concentrations of a large number of drugs. St. John's wort can decrease oral contraceptive levels by 13%–15%, resulting in bleeding or unplanned pregnancy; women should use an additional or nonhormonal form of birth control.

EVIDENCE AND CLINICAL PEARLS:
- Adult studies have been mixed, but most have reported St. John's wort is more effective than placebo, likely as effective as low-dose TCAs and SSRIs in milder forms of depression.
- No quality studies in pediatric depression. One randomized trial in pediatric ADHD (n = 54) found no benefit of St. John's wort 300 mg TID over placebo.

FUN FACTS:
Although not indigenous to Australia and long considered a weed, St. John's wort is now grown as a cash crop, and Australia produces 20% of the world's supply. St. John's wort is so named because it blooms near June 24th, which is the birthday of John the Baptist. "Wort" is an old English word for plant.

BOTTOM LINE:
St. John's wort can be considered an option for short-term treatment of mild depression in adults, but for kids the evidence is weaker.

VITAMIN D Fact Sheet

PEDIATRIC AND ADULT FDA INDICATIONS:
None.

OFF-LABEL USES:
Depression.

DOSAGE FORMS:
Supplied over the counter as vitamin D2 and D3, as tablets, capsules, and softgels in "international units" (IU) dosing. We recommend D3: 1000 IU, 2000 IU, 5000 IU, 10,000 IU.

PEDIATRIC DOSAGE GUIDANCE:
Dosing guidelines vary. For depression, use 1000–2500 IU per day.

COST: $

SIDE EFFECTS:
- Most common: well-tolerated.
- Serious but rare: vitamin D toxicity. Osteoporosis with doses over 5000 IU per day, and dietary habits such as excessive consumption of carbonated beverages may exacerbate this risk.

MECHANISM, PHARMACOKINETICS, AND DRUG INTERACTIONS:
- Thought to play a role in brain plasticity, neuroimmunomodulation, and inflammation.
- Metabolized by liver and kidneys; t ½: 12–50 days (varies based on level, source, dose, obesity, race).
- No known significant interactions.

EVIDENCE AND CLINICAL PEARLS:
- Several meta-analyses have found no beneficial effects of vitamin D supplementation in adults with depression. When studies were limited to depressed patients with both vitamin D insufficiency at baseline and adequate dosing of supplementation (>800 mg/day), statistically significant benefits were seen. No studies in pediatric depression.
- One small (n = 16) open-label study of vitamin D3 2000 IU daily in kids (6–17 years) with symptoms of mania showed improvement in mood symptoms.
- Sources of vitamin D include exposure to sunlight, dietary intake, and supplements.
- It's difficult to obtain sufficient daily needs from dietary intake alone. Two types of vitamin D are obtained from dietary sources: D2 (ergocalciferol) from plant sources such as mushrooms and soy milk and D3 (cholecalciferol) from animal sources such as raw fish, mackerel, and smoked salmon. D3 is approximately 3 times stronger than D2.
- The majority of vitamin D is produced through conversion of 7-dehydrocholesterol via ultraviolet B, after penetration of sunlight on the skin, to vitamin D3.
- Vitamin D is metabolized in the liver to 25-hydroxyvitamin D or 25(OH)D and then in the kidneys to its active form calcitriol, or 1,25-dihydroxyvitamin D. Labs will usually report 25(OH)D level with 30–60 ng/ml as normal range, 21–29 ng/ml as insufficiency, and <20 ng/ml as deficiency.

FUN FACT:
A number of things affect a person's vitamin D status, including distance from the equator, community air quality, skin color, and use of sunscreen.

BOTTOM LINE:
Vitamin D supplementation may be beneficial in adults with depression, but there is only minimal evidence in pediatric patients with mania. Reserve its use for those who have insufficiency, and have your patients take 1000–2000 IU daily.

Mood Stabilizers

The diagnosis of bipolar disorder in youth has shifted over time; once largely reserved for post-pubertal adolescents, now it encompasses a larger age range, including preschool-aged children. With changes made in the DSM-5, more children may now fall into the category of disruptive mood dysregulation disorder (DMDD) instead of the catchall diagnosis of bipolar disorder NOS. It is important to note the gravity of making a clear diagnosis prior to considering medication management, as the treatment options leave much to be desired.

The largest study examining the efficacy of mood stabilizers for children and adolescents is the Treatment of Early Age Mania (TEAM) study, which compared risperidone, lithium, and valproic acid in a randomized controlled trial of 279 subjects never treated with mood stabilizers. Risperidone was found to be more effective than either lithium or valproic acid in the treatment of an active manic or mixed episode. There are some data that support the use of lamotrigine for bipolar depression in teens.

Mainstay options are the classic mood stabilizers. These include lithium and anticonvulsants such as valproic acid, lamotrigine, carbamazepine, and antipsychotics.

- Lithium is effective for mania and yields a demonstrated reduction in suicidal behaviors and suicide rates when compared to placebo. Disadvantages include a number of side effects, a narrow therapeutic window, congenital risks in the first trimester, and potential longer-term harm to kidney function.

- Valproic acid is also effective for mania, but try to avoid it in females of childbearing age, both because it is teratogenic and because it increases the risk of polycystic ovary syndrome (PCOS).

- Lamotrigine could be considered for maintenance therapy; however, downsides include the slow titration schedule, increased risk of rash in children, and limited pediatric data.

- Carbamazepine would not be considered a first-line option, but it has a couple of open-label studies that showed improvements in depression and mania.

- Second-generation antipsychotics are increasingly being considered as first-line options for pediatric bipolar disorder. Despite serious metabolic side effects, their ease of use and rapidly accumulating evidence supporting effectiveness works in their favor. Lurasidone recently obtained FDA approval for pediatric bipolar depression, joining the ranks of asenapine for acute mania/mixed episodes, as well as risperidone, aripiprazole, olanzapine, and quetiapine. For detailed information about specific agents, refer to the antipsychotics chapter.

SIDE EFFECTS AND CLASS WARNINGS

- Class warning of suicidality: All antiepileptics include this warning based on an analysis of anticonvulsant trials for a wide range of diagnoses, which demonstrated an increased risk of suicidal thoughts or behaviors from 1 week through 24 weeks of treatment compared to placebo. This risk was also noted to be higher in patients with a seizure disorder.

- Black box warning of lithium toxicity, with monitoring required for lithium levels given the narrow therapeutic window. Target levels range from 0.6–1.2 mEq/L, although mild toxicity can also occur within the normal range. Toxicity can involve confusion, ataxia, tremors, myoclonus, fasciculations, GI symptoms, renal symptoms, and arrhythmia.

- Hypersensitivity reactions: Some antiepileptic medications, including valproic acid and lamotrigine, include a warning for DRESS (drug rash with eosinophilia and systemic symptoms)/multi-organ hypersensitivity reactions, which may be life-threatening or fatal. Symptoms may include fever, lymphadenopathy, or rash. Skin precautions are important (eg, sun protection).

- Abrupt discontinuation of anticonvulsant medications may lead to rebound seizures and should generally be avoided if possible.

- GI adverse effects are common with lithium and anticonvulsants. Fatigue and sedation, as well as cognitive side effects, can occur with these medications. Drowsy driving is a particular hazard.

- Metabolic side effects associated with weight gain may occur with antipsychotics and mood stabilizers, with the exception of lamotrigine and topiramate.

- Menstrual changes may occur with lithium and several anticonvulsants.

TABLE 8: Mood Stabilizers

Generic Name (Brand Name) Year FDA Approved for Bipolar Disorder or Mania [G] denotes generic availability	Relevant FDA Indication(s) (Pediatric FDA approval bolded)	Available Strengths (mg)	Usual Pediatric Dosage Range (mg)	Comments
Carbamazepine [G] (Carbatrol, Epitol, Equetro, Tegretol, Tegretol XR) 2004	Bipolar disorder (Equetro: acute mania)	CH: 100, 200 IR: 100, 200, 300, 400 ER: 100, 200, 300, 400 Oral solution: 100 mg/5 mL	200–1200	Open-label data only, but safety data in kids for seizures
Lamotrigine [G] (Lamictal, Lamictal CD, Lamictal ODT, Lamictal XR) 2003	Bipolar disorder (maintenance)	IR: 5, 25, 50, 100, 150, 200, 250 CH: 2, 5, 25 ODT: 25, 50, 100, 200 ER: 25, 50, 100, 200, 250, 300	100–400	Open-label data; caution: rash risk greater in kids
Lithium [G] (Lithobid) 1970	**Acute mania Bipolar maintenance (12–17 yrs)**	IR: 150, 300, 600 ER: 300, 450 Oral solution: 300 mg/5 mL	300–2400	FDA indication in kids; first-line choice
Oxcarbazepine [G] (Trileptal, Oxtellar XR) 2000*	Not approved for any bipolar indication	IR: 150, 300, 600 ER: 150, 300, 600 Oral suspension: 300 mg/5 mL	600–2400	No positive efficacy data to support use in kids, but safety data in kids with seizures
Valproic acid [G] (Depakene, Depakote, Depakote ER, Depakote Sprinkles) 1995	Bipolar disorder (acute mania)	IR: 250 Liquid: 250 mg/5 mL DR: 125, 250, 500 ER: 250, 500	500–2000	Open-label data only, but safety data in kids for seizures; first-line choice

CH = chewable, IR = immediate release, ER = extended release, ODT = orally disintegrating tablet, DR = delayed release

*oxcarbazepine FDA approved for seizure disorder

CARBAMAZEPINE (Tegretol) Fact Sheet [G]

PEDIATRIC FDA INDICATIONS:
Seizure disorders.

ADULT FDA INDICATIONS:
Seizures; trigeminal neuralgia; bipolar disorder (Equetro: acute mania).

OFF-LABEL USES:
Bipolar maintenance; impulse control disorders; violence and aggression; migraine prophylaxis.

DOSAGE FORMS:
- **Chewable tablets (G):** 100 mg, 200 mg (scored).
- **Tablets (Tegretol, Epitol, G):** 100 mg, 200 mg, 300 mg, 400 mg (scored).
- **ER tablets (Tegretol XR, G):** 100 mg, 200 mg, 400 mg.
- **ER capsules (Equetro, Carbatrol, G):** 100 mg, 200 mg, 300 mg.
- **Oral solution (Tegretol, G):** 100 mg/5 mL.

PEDIATRIC DOSAGE GUIDANCE:
- Age <6 years: Start 10–20 mg/kg/day divided BID–QID, increase by 5–10 mg/kg/day in weekly intervals; max 35 mg/kg/day.
- Age 6–12 years: Start 100 mg BID, increase by 100 mg/day in weekly intervals; max 1000 mg/day in divided doses.
- Age >12 years: Start 200 mg BID and gradually ↑ by 200 mg/day in weekly intervals; max 1200 mg/day.
- Dosing is the same for IR and ER versions of carbamazepine; both are BID.

MONITORING: CBC, electrolytes (sodium), LFTs, pregnancy test, serum level, HLA-B*1502 (Asians), ECG if cardiac risk.

COST: IR: $; ER: $$

SIDE EFFECTS:
- Most common: dizziness, somnolence, nausea, headache. (ER versions may cause fewer side effects in some patients, but the evidence is not clear.)
- Serious but rare: hematologic abnormalities including agranulocytosis, aplastic anemia, neutropenia, leukopenia, thrombocytopenia, and pancytopenia reported; hepatic complications including slight increases in hepatic enzymes, cholestatic and hepatocellular jaundice, hepatitis (and, rarely, hepatic failure), hyponatremia, SIADH; rash (5%–10%), including exfoliation, reported. Severe reactions, including toxic epidermal necrolysis and Stevens-Johnson syndrome, are rare but can be fatal.

MECHANISM, PHARMACOKINETICS, AND DRUG INTERACTIONS:
- Sodium channel blocker. Metabolized primarily through CYP3A4; t ½: 15 hours (initially 25–65 hours, but induces its own metabolism over approximately 2–4 weeks with each dosage change and then stabilizes).
- Highly significant interactions: potent inducer of CYP1A2, CYP2B6, CYP2C19, CYP2C8, CYP2C9, CYP3A4, P-glycoprotein; medications significantly metabolized through these pathways may become subtherapeutic; caution in patients taking strong CYP3A4 inducers or inhibitors that can affect carbamazepine levels.
- Avoid use with oral contraceptives (lowers levels/unplanned pregnancies) and clozapine (agranulocytosis).

EVIDENCE AND CLINICAL PEARLS:
- Pediatric bipolar data limited to open-label studies with only modest response rates (38%–44%).
- Therapeutic level: 4 mcg/mL–12 mcg/mL in seizure disorders. No correlation in bipolar disorder—best dosed clinically. Check levels 5 days and a few weeks after changes due to induction of enzymes that affect levels.
- Avoid use if variant HLA-B*1502 allele (Asian): risk of Stevens-Johnson syndrome/toxic epidermal necrolysis.

FUN FACT:
May cause false-positive TCA screen as its chemical structure contains the tricyclic nucleus common to TCAs.

BOTTOM LINE:
Not a first-line treatment for bipolar disorder in kids due to limited data, side effect profile, and high likelihood of significant interactions. Used in kids for seizure disorders, so we have some basis of safety information. Equetro is FDA-approved for bipolar disorder (in adults), but other cheaper formulations give similar results.

LAMOTRIGINE (Lamictal) Fact Sheet [G]

PEDIATRIC FDA INDICATIONS:
Seizures.

ADULT FDA INDICATIONS:
Bipolar disorder (maintenance) in adults; seizures.

OFF-LABEL USES:
Bipolar depression; neuropathic pain; major depression; borderline personality disorder.

DOSAGE FORMS:
- **Tablets (G):** 5 mg, 25 mg, 50 mg, 100 mg, 150 mg, 200 mg, 250 mg (scored).
- **Chewable tablets (Lamictal CD, G):** 2 mg, 5 mg, 25 mg.
- **Orally disintegrating tablets (Lamictal ODT, G):** 25 mg, 50 mg, 100 mg, 200 mg.
- **ER tablets (Lamictal XR, G):** 25 mg, 50 mg, 100 mg, 200 mg, 250 mg, 300 mg.

PEDIATRIC DOSAGE GUIDANCE (BASED ON DOSING IN KIDS WITH SEIZURES):
- Bipolar disorder: Start 25 mg QD for 2 weeks, ↑ to 50 mg QD for 2 weeks, then 100 mg QD; max 200 mg/day.
- Patients on valproate: Start 25 mg QOD (every other day) for 2 weeks, ↑ to 25 mg QD for 2 weeks, then 50 mg QD; max 100 mg/day (VPA doubles lamotrigine levels).
- Dosing is the same with all versions of lamotrigine.

MONITORING: No specific monitoring of note.

COST: IR: $; ER: $$$

SIDE EFFECTS:
- Most common: dizziness, headache, nausea, sedation, benign rash (7%).
- Rare, potentially life-threatening skin reactions (black box warning) including Stevens-Johnson Syndrome/toxic epidermal necrolysis, requiring hospitalization reported; incidence higher in pediatric patients; increased in co-administration with valproic acid, higher-than-recommended starting doses, and exceeding of recommended dose titration. Other risk factors include infections (herpes simplex, herpes zoster, HIV, hepatitis A, pneumonia), immunocompromise, and HLA-B 1502 (common in India, China, and Southeast Asia). Usually occurs before 8 weeks with isolated cases beyond 8 weeks and without risk factors. Discontinue at first sign of rash and do not reinitiate unless rash is clearly not drug-related; rare cases of hemophagocytic lymphohistiocytosis (HLH), and angioedema reported.

MECHANISM, PHARMACOKINETICS, AND DRUG INTERACTIONS:
- Sodium channel blocker. Metabolism primarily hepatic (non-P450); t ½: 25–33 hours (with VPA 48–70 hours; with carbamazepine 13–14 hours).
- Enzyme-inducing medications (eg, carbamazepine) and hormonal contraceptives decrease lamotrigine levels; lamotrigine may need to be increased (2-fold). Gradual increases of lamotrigine levels may occur during the inactive "pill-free" week. Lamotrigine may decrease hormonal contraceptives (estrogens more than progestins); consider alternative birth control methods. Valproic acid may double lamotrigine levels, necessitating much slower titration or dosage adjustments (as above).

EVIDENCE AND CLINICAL PEARLS:
- One open-label response: monotherapy in pediatric bipolar disorder, 54% for manic symptoms.
- For maintenance in adult bipolar disorder; prophylaxis of depression. Not useful in acute episodes.
- If stopped/missed >5 half-lives (see above), restart with initial dosing protocol to minimize rash risk.
- FDA warning: rare cases of HLH, a life-threatening immune reaction. Refer immediately for persistent fever (>101°F); rash; pain, tenderness, or swelling in the area of the liver; swollen lymph nodes; jaundice; unusual bleeding; and nervous system problems such as seizures, trouble walking, or visual difficulties.

FUN FACT:
The first FDA-approved drug for bipolar disorder in adults (not just acute mania) since lithium, a drug approved more than 30 years earlier (2003 for lamotrigine; 1970 for lithium).

BOTTOM LINE:
Not for first-line use for most kids due to limited data (open-label studies only) and increased relative risk of rash in pediatric population.

LITHIUM (Lithobid) Fact Sheet [G]

PEDIATRIC FDA INDICATIONS:
Acute mania; bipolar disorder maintenance (12–17 years).

ADULT FDA INDICATIONS:
Acute mania; bipolar disorder maintenance.

OFF-LABEL USES:
Bipolar depression; treatment-resistant depression; neutropenia; vascular headache.

DOSAGE FORMS:
- **Capsules (lithium carbonate, G):** 150 mg, 300 mg, 600 mg.
- **Tablets (lithium carbonate, G):** 300 mg.
- **ER tablets: Lithobid, G:** 300 mg; **Eskalith CR, G:** 450 mg (scored).
- **Oral solution (lithium citrate, G):** 300 mg/5 mL.

PEDIATRIC DOSAGE GUIDANCE (DOSING SAME FOR IR AND ER VERSIONS; BOTH ARE BID):
- <30 kg: Start 10 mg/kg/day divided BID–QID, increase by 5–10 mg/kg/day in weekly intervals to target dose 15–40 mg/kg/day divided TID–QID; max 60 mg/kg/day.
- >30 kg: Start 10–20 mg/kg/day divided BID–QID, increase by 10 mg/kg/day in weekly intervals to target dose 15–40 mg/kg/day divided TID–QID; max 60 mg/kg/day.
- Adolescents: Start 600–900 mg/day divided BID–TID, increase by 300 mg/day in weekly intervals to target dose 900–1200 mg/day divided TID–QID; max 2400 mg/day.

MONITORING: TSH, BUN/creatinine, CBC, basic metabolic panel, weight, pregnancy test, serum drug level, ECG if cardiac disease or older patient.

COST: IR, ER: $

SIDE EFFECTS:
- Most common: nausea/diarrhea (take with meals, split dosing, switch to ER), fine tremor (lower dose or use propranolol), polyuria/excessive thirst (dose all at bedtime), memory problems, weight gain, hypothyroidism (7%–8%; 9 times more common in women), acne or worsening psoriasis, benign increase in WBC.
- Serious but rare: Chronic use may result in diminished renal concentrating ability (nephrogenic diabetes insipidus); usually reverses when discontinued, or treat with hydrochlorothiazide 25 mg–50 mg/day or amiloride 5 mg–10 mg twice daily. Cardiac: bradycardia, cardiac arrhythmia, flattened or inverted T waves, sinus node dysfunction may occur rarely; normal pressure hydrocephalus characterized by loss of bladder control, delirium, and ataxia (wet, wild, and wobbly). These side effects require immediate discontinuation and possibly dialysis to extract lithium from the patient.

MECHANISM, PHARMACOKINETICS, AND DRUG INTERACTIONS:
- Alters neuronal sodium transport.
- Eliminated by kidneys; t ½: 18–24 hours.
- Drugs that increase lithium levels: "**N**o **ACE** in the **H**ole" (**N**SAIDs, **ACE** inhibitors, and **H**CTZ); excess sweating can increase levels; low-sodium diet may increase lithium levels. Caffeine may decrease levels.

EVIDENCE AND CLINICAL PEARLS:
- Four open-label trials of lithium in pediatric bipolar disorder suggest efficacy; only 1 of these was monotherapy (with a 38% response rate). More recent double-blind studies did not show benefit over placebo in mania, yet lithium is FDA-indicated for kids >12 years.
- Check lithium level, TSH/T4, BUN/Cr, CBC, BMP, electrolytes after 1 week of treatment, at 1–2 months, then every 6–12 months. Target levels for acute mania: 0.8–1.2 mEq/L; maintenance: 0.6–1.0 mEq/L; toxicity >1.5 mEq/L, but may see signs at lower levels. Levels should be drawn 12 hours after a dose; steady state generally reached after 5 days.
- An increase or decrease of 300 mg/day will change serum level by roughly 0.25±0.1 mEq/L.
- Dehydration: Use with caution in patients with significant fluid loss (protracted sweating, diarrhea, or prolonged fever); temporary reduction or discontinuation may be necessary.
- Shown to have anti-suicide effects in bipolar and unipolar mood disorders in adults.

FUN FACTS:
The soft drink 7-Up was originally called "Bib-Label Lithiated Lemon-Lime Soda" and contained lithium until 1950.

BOTTOM LINE:
Although clinicians often try other medications first due to both the relative complexity of managing lithium as well as bias from the public, lithium, along with several second-generation antipsychotics, is FDA-indicated and considered first-line for treating pediatric bipolar disorder. Although it is not free from side effects, most common effects can be managed quite well.

OXCARBAZEPINE (Trileptal) Fact Sheet [G]

PEDIATRIC FDA INDICATIONS:
Seizures.

ADULT FDA INDICATIONS:
Seizure disorders.

OFF-LABEL USES:
Bipolar disorder.

DOSAGE FORMS:
- **Tablets (G):** 150 mg, 300 mg, 600 mg (scored).
- **Oral suspension (G):** 300 mg/5 mL.
- **ER tablets (Oxtellar XR):** 150 mg, 300 mg, 600 mg.

PEDIATRIC DOSAGE GUIDANCE:
- Start 8–10 mg/kg/day divided BID, increase by 5 mg/kg/day in weekly intervals to usual 600–900 mg/day divided BID; max 2400 mg/day.
- No data on use of XR for bipolar disorder; caution as higher doses of XR likely needed when converting from IR to XR (not interchangeable on dose-for-dose basis).

MONITORING: Electrolytes (sodium), HLA-B*1502 in Asians.

COST: IR: $; ER: $$$$

SIDE EFFECTS:
- Most common: dizziness, somnolence, headache, ataxia, nausea, vomiting.
- Serious but rare: potentially serious, sometimes fatal, dermatologic reactions (eg, Stevens-Johnson syndrome, toxic epidermal necrolysis) reported; monitor for skin reactions. Rare cases of anaphylaxis and angioedema reported, even after initial dosing; permanently discontinue should symptoms occur.
- Use caution in patients with previous hypersensitivity to carbamazepine (cross-sensitivity occurs in 25%–30%). Clinically significant hyponatremia (serum sodium <125 mmol/L) may develop (1%–3%; higher rate than with carbamazepine); monitor serum sodium, particularly during the first 3 months of therapy, especially in patients at risk for hyponatremia.

MECHANISM, PHARMACOKINETICS, AND DRUG INTERACTIONS:
- Sodium channel blocker and neuronal membrane stabilizer.
- Metabolized primarily through CYP450; potent inducer of CYP3A4 and inhibitor of CYP2C19; t ½: 2 hours (9 hours for active metabolite).
- No auto-induction of metabolism and fewer interactions than with carbamazepine. Avoid concomitant use with medications metabolized by CYP3A4 since oxcarbazepine may reduce their levels. Reduces efficacy of oral contraceptives; try nonhormonal measures.

EVIDENCE AND CLINICAL PEARLS:
- In a double-blind study in pediatric mania, it was not statistically better than placebo.
- Oxcarbazepine is the 10-keto analog of carbamazepine (its "chemical cousin"); it is thought of as a gentler carbamazepine due to its more favorable side effect and drug interaction profile.
- Not bioequivalent to carbamazepine. Increase total daily dose by 20%–30% if switching from carbamazepine to oxcarbazepine.
- Screen and avoid using in patients of Asian descent who have HLA-B*1502 allele; risk of Stevens-Johnson syndrome and/or toxic epidermal necrolysis. Avoid use in such patients.

FUN FACT:
Synthesized in 1965, oxcarbazepine appeared on the US market in 2000. In 2010, Novartis pled guilty to marketing it for non-FDA-approved uses, eg, neuropathic pain and bipolar disorder.

BOTTOM LINE:
Compared to carbamazepine, oxcarbazepine poses less concern for drug interactions and for hepatic or hematologic toxicities; it also does not require serum level monitoring. However, due to lack of efficacy data in pediatric bipolar disorder, we do not recommend its general use for that disorder. Still, some clinicians use oxcarbazepine to try to reduce irritability in a wider range of clinical circumstances. It is reserved for second-line use after lithium and valproic acid.

VALPROIC ACID (Depakote) Fact Sheet [G]

PEDIATRIC FDA INDICATIONS:
Seizures.

ADULT FDA INDICATIONS:
Seizures; bipolar disorder (acute mania); migraine prophylaxis.

OFF-LABEL USES:
Bipolar maintenance; impulse control disorders; violence and aggression.

DOSAGE FORMS:
- **Capsules (valproic acid, G):** 250 mg.
- **Oral liquid (Depakene, G):** 250 mg/5 mL.
- **Tablets (delayed release) (Depakote, G):** 125 mg, 250 mg, 500 mg.
- **Capsules (delayed release) (Depakote Sprinkles, G):** 125 mg.
- **ER tablets (Depakote ER, G):** 250 mg, 500 mg.

PEDIATRIC DOSAGE GUIDANCE:
- Start 15 mg/kg/day divided BID–TID, increase by 5–10 mg/kg/day in weekly intervals; max 60 mg/kg/day. Typical dosing range in kids is 500–2000 mg/day divided BID–TID.
- When converting from regular Depakote to Depakote ER, be aware that patients will get about 20% less valproic acid with the ER formulation.

MONITORING: LFTs, CBC for platelets, lipids, pregnancy test, weight, serum drug level, ammonia in patients with confusion, and amylase and lipase when pancreatitis is suspected.

COST: DR: $; ER: $$

SIDE EFFECTS:
- Most common: somnolence, nausea, fatigue, dizziness, hair loss, tremor, thrombocytopenia (up to 24% of patients; dose-related; reversible).
- Serious but rare: hepatotoxicity—rare idiosyncratic reaction, not dose-related; most cases occur within 3 months; risk factors: age <2 years, multiple anticonvulsants, and presence of neurologic disease in addition to epilepsy. Asymptomatic elevations of liver enzymes may occur, not necessarily associated with hepatic dysfunction. Pancreatitis (rare but potentially fatal). Polycystic ovary syndrome (PCOS) in about 10% of women. Hyperammonemia, encephalopathy (sometimes fatal) reported and may present with normal liver enzymes.

MECHANISM, PHARMACOKINETICS, AND DRUG INTERACTIONS:
- Sodium channel blocker.
- Metabolized primarily by liver with only minimal (10%) role of CYP450 enzymes (2A6, 2B6, 2C9); t ½: 9–16 hours.
- VPA causes ↑ levels of lamotrigine and risk for rash. Taking with topiramate can lead to encephalopathy.

EVIDENCE AND CLINICAL PEARLS:
- Significantly more data in pediatric bipolar than other agents, with 8 open-label (average response rate: 43%) and 3 double-blind studies, 1 of which did not separate from placebo.
- Once steady-state levels reached (within 2–4 days of initiation or dose adjustment), trough serum levels should be drawn just before the next dose (ER/DR preparations) or before the morning dose (for immediate release preparations).
- Valproate often reduces available carnitine, which is needed for cell transport physiology. This results in elevated ammonia levels, creating fatigue, confusion, and other symptoms of metabolic stress. Carnitine can be very safely replaced using a minimum twice-daily dosing of carnitine in 330 mg capsules (can be opened, but contents have a strong odor) and titrating up based on repeat laboratory studies.

FUN FACT:
Valproic acid was first synthesized in 1882 by B. S. Burton as an analogue of valeric acid, found naturally in valerian.

BOTTOM LINE:
Along with lithium, valproate is a first-line antimanic agent for acute manic episodes in kids. In girls of child-bearing age, consider risk of PCOS as well as risk of congenital malformation and ensure adequate contraception (ideally IUD or depot contraceptive).

Substance Use Medications

The primary treatment of substance use disorders involves behavioral therapies. Although substance use medications are likely effective in adolescents, none are currently FDA-approved for this age group, with the exception of buprenorphine for adolescents age 16 and up. Any adult indications and dosing recommendations should therefore be used as a guide. It's also important to address comorbid mental health conditions, specifically ADHD, because treating such kids with stimulants may decrease the risk of substance use, according to some studies.

NICOTINE USE DISORDERS

Nicotine replacement therapies are available in many forms and may help with weaning adolescents off of nicotine; however, some clinicians argue that despite harm reduction benefits, continued nicotine use in any form can be harmful to the developing brain. Obtain a thorough history to calculate daily nicotine use, using the guideline that 1 pack per day = 21 mg. The patch should be placed in different positions at the same time each day to avoid skin irritation, and used for 1–2 months, then tapered every 1–2 months as tolerated. Take note that nicotine patches and gum are available over the counter for adults only, so you'll have to write out a prescription for those under 18. Bupropion is effective for smoking cessation in adults, and though we don't have sufficient data for adolescents, we know that bupropion is generally a safe medication for this age group. Varenicline can help decrease cravings in adults, but data on efficacy and safety for smoking cessation in adolescents is lacking.

ALCOHOL USE DISORDERS

While not often used in adolescents, 3 medications are approved in adults for alcohol use. Acamprosate can be useful in reducing cravings and for maintaining abstinence through its modulating effects on the glutamate system. Disulfiram inhibits the breakdown of alcohol by inhibiting alcohol dehydrogenase, which leads to headaches, flushing, nausea, and tachycardia in those who drink while taking the medication. Disulfiram cannot be started until 12–36 hours after the last drink, and adherence can be low—so, given the impulsivity of adolescents who are drinking, disulfiram is unlikely to be appropriate in most patients. Naltrexone acts on an opioid receptor to blunt the pleasurable effects of alcohol as well as decrease cravings. Topiramate, though not FDA-approved for this use, is effective in reducing alcohol craving in adults.

OPIOID USE DISORDERS

Naltrexone is an opioid antagonist that you can start after your patient completes detox, and it works by preventing the opioid from causing euphoria. It is the least burdensome medication that can be used for the treatment of opioid use. Buprenorphine has a few adolescent studies that demonstrate efficacy in decreasing withdrawal and cravings. Monthly office-based maintenance treatment is available, which provides more flexibility than methadone maintenance. Methadone is an opioid agonist that can be used as a substitute for other opiates, but it has limited effect in achieving sobriety. Some states allow older adolescents that have failed other treatments to receive methadone treatment with the consent of their guardian. It comes with the onerous requirement of presenting daily to the methadone clinic in order to receive a dose, which can be very limiting with regard to vocational, academic, and family schedules. Finally, naloxone is now more readily available to families and emergency service personnel to reverse opioid overdose and prevent deaths.

OTHER DRUGS

There are currently no FDA-approved medications in adults or adolescents to address cocaine, benzodiazepine, methamphetamine, or cannabis use, so we haven't included fact sheets for medications addressing these specific issues. However, you might find the Carlat Psychiatry Guidebook, *Addiction Treatment* by Michael Weaver, MD, a useful resource.

TABLE 9: Substance Use and Dependence Medications

Generic Name (Brand Name) Year FDA Approved (Rx status) [G] denotes generic availability	Relevant FDA Indication(s)	Available Strengths (mg)	Usual Adult Dosage Range (mg)
Acamprosate [G] (Campral) 2004 (Rx)	Alcohol	333	666 TID
Buprenorphine [G] (Buprenex, Butrans) 2002 (C-III)	Opiate (16+ yrs)	2, 8 SL 0.3 mg/mL inj (used for pain) 5, 7.5, 10, 15, 20 mcg/h patch (used for pain)	8 QD–16 QD
Buprenorphine subdermal implant (Probuphine) 2016 (C-III)	Opiate	Each implant contains equivalent of 80 mg of buprenorphine	Four implants x1, delivering dose up to 6 months
Buprenorphine and Naloxone [G] (Bunavail, Suboxone, Zubsolv) 2002 (C-III) Generic available for 2/0.5, 8/2 mg SL tablets and film strips only	Opiate (16+ yrs)	2.1/0.3, 4.2/0.7, 6.3/1 buccal film (Bunavail) 2/0.5, 4/1, 8/2, 12/3 SL film strips (Suboxone, generic) 2/0.5, 8/2 SL tabs (generic only) 1.4/0.36, 2.9/0.71, 5.7/1.4, 8.6/2.1, 11.4/2.9 SL tabs (Zubsolv)	4–24 QD
Bupropion SR [G] (Zyban) 1997 (Rx)	Smoking	150	150 QAM–150 BID
Disulfiram [G] (Antabuse) 1951 (Rx)	Alcohol	250, 500	125 QPM–500 QPM
Methadone [G] (Dolophine, Methadose) 1947 (C-II)	Opiate	5, 10, 40 10 mg/mL, 10 mg/5 mL, 5 mg/5 mL oral liquid	20 QD–120 QD
Naloxone (Evzio, Narcan Nasal Spray) 2014 (auto-injector) 2015 (intranasal) (Rx)	Emergency opioid overdose rescue	2 mg/0.4 mL autoinjector 2 mg/0.1 mL, 4 mg/0.1 mL intranasal	IV/IM/SC: Infants and children ≤5 years or ≤20 kg: 0.1 mg/kg/dose. Children >5 years or >20 kg and adolescents: 2 mg/dose. Intranasal: 4 mg x1, repeat every 2–3 minutes.
Naltrexone [G] (ReVia) 1984 (Rx)	Alcohol, opiate	50	25 QD–50 QD
Naltrexone ER (Vivitrol) 2006 (Rx)	Alcohol, opiate	380	380 Q 4wk
Nicotine inhaled (Nicotrol Inhaler) 1997 (Rx)	Smoking	4 mg delivered/cartridge	6–16 cartridges per day

Substance Use Medications

Generic Name (Brand Name) Year FDA Approved (Rx status) [G] denotes generic availability	Relevant FDA Indication(s)	Available Strengths (mg)	Usual Adult Dosage Range (mg)
Nicotine nasal spray (Nicotrol NS) 1996 (Rx)	Smoking	0.5 mg delivered/spray	1–2 sprays/hour PRN
Nicotine polacrilex [G] (Nicorette Gum, others) 1992 (OTC; Rx if <18 yrs)	Smoking	2, 4	1 piece PRN up to 24/day
Nicotine polacrilex [G] (Nicorette Lozenge, others) 2009 (OTC; Rx if <18 yrs)	Smoking	2, 4	1 piece PRN up to 20/day
Nicotine transdermal [G] (Habitrol, Nicoderm CQ) 1991 (OTC; Rx if <18 yrs)	Smoking	7, 14, 21/24 hours	14–21 QD
Varenicline (Chantix) 2006 (Rx)	Smoking	0.5, 1	0.5 QD–1 BID

ACAMPROSATE (Campral) Fact Sheet [G]

PEDIATRIC FDA INDICATIONS:
None.

ADULT FDA INDICATIONS:
Alcohol dependence.

OFF-LABEL USES:
None.

DOSAGE FORMS:
Delayed release tablets (G): 333 mg.

DOSAGE GUIDANCE (ADULT):
Start 666 mg TID. Give 333 mg TID in patients with renal impairment.

MONITORING: BUN/creatinine.

COST: $$$

SIDE EFFECTS:
- Most common: diarrhea (dose-related, transient), flatulence, weakness, peripheral edema, insomnia, anxiety.
- Serious but rare: acute renal failure reported in a few cases; suicidal ideation, attempts, and completions rare but greater than with placebo in studies.

MECHANISM, PHARMACOKINETICS, AND DRUG INTERACTIONS:
- Mechanism of action is not fully defined; it appears to work by promoting a balance between the excitatory and inhibitory neurotransmitters, glutamate and GABA, respectively (GABA and glutamate activities appear to be disrupted in alcohol dependence).
- Not metabolized, cleared as unchanged drug by kidneys; t ½: 20–33 hours.
- There are no significant drug interactions.

EVIDENCE AND CLINICAL PEARLS:
- Clinically, acamprosate has demonstrated efficacy in more than 25 placebo-controlled trials in adults, and it has generally been found to be more effective than placebo in reducing risk of returning to any drinking and increasing the cumulative duration of abstinence. However, in reducing heavy drinking, acamprosate appears to be no better than placebo.
- Clinical data in adolescents with alcohol use disorder is limited but promising. There are additional studies in children with autism and fragile X syndrome that have found acamprosate to be generally safe and well-tolerated in the pediatric population.
- Acamprosate can be used with naltrexone or disulfiram (different mechanism of action), although the combination with naltrexone may not increase efficacy per available studies.
- Approved by the FDA in 2004, but it has been used in France and other countries since 1989.
- Does not eliminate or treat symptoms of alcohol withdrawal. Usually prescribed for maintenance of abstinence; may continue even if patient relapses with alcohol.
- Taking with food is not necessary, but it may help compliance to do so.
- Compared to naltrexone and disulfiram, acamprosate is unique in that it is not metabolized by the liver and is not impacted by alcohol use, so it can be administered to patients with hepatitis or liver disease and to patients who continue drinking alcohol.

FUN FACT:
Each 333 mg tablet contains 33 mg of elemental calcium (because it is available as acamprosate calcium salt).

BOTTOM LINE:
Acamprosate and naltrexone show similar reduced rates of relapse, but acamprosate is associated with more diarrhea, while naltrexone is associated with more nausea, fatigue, and somnolence; acamprosate is preferred in patients with hepatic impairment. Limited data in children, but seems to be well-tolerated.

BUPRENORPHINE (Buprenex, Probuphine, Sublocade) Fact Sheet [G]

PEDIATRIC FDA INDICATIONS:
Pain (2+ years).

ADULT FDA INDICATIONS (16+ YEARS):
Opioid dependence, induction; moderate-severe pain (Belbuca, Buprenex, Butrans); opioid dependence, maintenance (Probuphine, Sublocade).

OFF-LABEL USES:
None.

DOSAGE FORMS:
- **SL tablets (G):** 2 mg, 8 mg (scored).
- **Injection (G):** 0.3 mg/mL (used for pain).
- **Transdermal patch (Butrans):** 5 mcg/h, 7.5 mcg/h, 10 mcg/h, 15 mcg/h, 20 mcg/h (used for pain).
- **Subdermal implant (Probuphine):** Each implant contains the equivalent of 80 mg of buprenorphine.
- **Extended release injection (Sublocade):** 100 mg/0.5 mL, 300 mg/1.5 mL prefilled syringes.

DOSAGE GUIDANCE (16+ YEARS):
- Start 2 mg–8 mg SL day 1; then 8 mg–16 mg SL QD (usual induction dose range is 12 mg–16 mg/day and accomplished over 3–4 days). Begin at least 4 hours after last use of heroin or other short-acting opioids and when first signs of withdrawal appear. If an opioid-dependent patient is not in sufficient withdrawal, introduction of buprenorphine may precipitate withdrawal due to its partial agonist effect. Other than implant, not for maintenance treatment; patients should be switched to the buprenorphine/naloxone combination for maintenance and unsupervised therapy.
- Patients stable on ≤8 mg/day for at least 3 months may convert to implants, available as four 1-inch flexible rods that are surgically implanted inside the upper arm and will deliver a low-level dose of buprenorphine for up to 6 months.
- Patients with moderate to severe opioid use disorder and stabilized with SL or buccal buprenorphine for >7 days may convert to monthly injections. Start 300 mg monthly for 2 months, then 100 mg monthly maintenance. Some patients may require higher doses.

MONITORING: LFTs.

COST: SL: $$$; implant: $$$$$; pricing for monthly injection not yet determined

SIDE EFFECTS:
- Most common: headache, pain, insomnia, nausea, anxiety; surgical site pain, itching, redness (Probuphine).
- Serious but rare: hepatitis reported rarely, ranging from transient, asymptomatic transaminase elevations to hepatic failure; in many cases, patients had preexisting hepatic dysfunction. QT prolongation with higher doses of transdermal.

MECHANISM, PHARMACOKINETICS, AND DRUG INTERACTIONS:
- Opioid agonist (delta and mu receptors) and antagonist (kappa receptors).
- Metabolized primarily through CYP3A4; t ½: 24–48 hours.
- Avoid concomitant use with opiate analgesics: diminished pain control. Additive effects with CNS depressants. CYP3A4 inhibitors and inducers may affect levels of buprenorphine.

EVIDENCE AND CLINICAL PEARLS:
- Adult response rates over 6 months similar between implant and SL tablets (63% and 64%, respectively). Convenient and less likely to be abused or resold illicitly. Disadvantages: complications from insertion and removal, and some patients may still need oral buprenorphine. Implants and injection offer alternatives for some patients, but these have only been studied in adults thus far.
- C-III controlled substance. Prescribing of SL tablets for opioid dependence is limited to physicians who have met qualification criteria and have received a DEA number specific to buprenorphine (see www.buprenorphine.samhsa.gov).
- Initially, each approved doctor could treat only 10 patients, but the law was modified to alleviate bottleneck treatment access; now each physician can treat up to 100 patients and after 1 year can become eligible to treat up to 275.
- Binds to various opioid receptors, producing agonism at delta receptors, partial agonism at mu receptors, and antagonism at kappa receptors (opioid agonist-antagonist).

FUN FACT:
Other subcutaneous implants currently in development include medications that will treat schizophrenia, breast cancer, photosensitivity, and Parkinson's disease.

BOTTOM LINE:
Buprenorphine alone was previously preferred for initial (induction) phase of treatment, with buprenorphine/naloxone combination preferred for maintenance treatment (unsupervised administration). Currently, combination is favored for both induction and maintenance as this decreases any abuse or diversion potential. Studied and approved for ages ≥16.

BUPRENORPHINE/NALOXONE (Suboxone) Fact Sheet [G]

PEDIATRIC FDA INDICATIONS:
None.

ADULT FDA INDICATIONS (16+ YEARS):
Opioid dependence (induction and maintenance); approved for adolescents aged 16+.

OFF-LABEL USES:
None.

DOSAGE FORMS:
- **SL tablets (G):** 2/0.5 mg, 8/2 mg (scored).
- **SL film strips (Suboxone, G):** 2/0.5 mg, 4/1 mg, 8/2 mg, 12/3 mg.
- **SL tablets (Zubsolv):** 1.4/0.36 mg, 2.9/0.71 mg, 5.7/1.4 mg, 8.6/2.1 mg, 11.4/2.9 mg.
- **Buccal film (Bunavail):** 2.1/0.3 mg, 4.2/0.7 mg, 6.3/1 mg.

DOSAGE GUIDANCE (16+ YEARS):
- For induction, use strategy described in buprenorphine fact sheet. For maintenance, give combination product (Suboxone or [G]) daily in the equivalent buprenorphine dose on last day of induction; adjust dose in increments of 2 mg or 4 mg to a level that maintains treatment and suppresses opioid withdrawal symptoms (usually 4 mg–24 mg/day); max 32 mg/day.
- Zubsolv 5.7/1.4 mg SL tablet provides equivalent buprenorphine to a Suboxone 8/2 mg SL tablet.
- Bunavail 4.2/0.7 mg buccal film provides equivalent buprenorphine to a Suboxone 8/2 mg SL tablet.

MONITORING: LFTs.

COST: SL tablet, film: $$$$; Zubsolv, Bunavail: $$$$$

SIDE EFFECTS:
- Most common: headache, pain, vomiting, sweating.
- Serious but rare: hepatitis reported rarely, ranging from transient, asymptomatic transaminase elevations to hepatic failure; in many cases, patients had preexisting hepatic dysfunction.

MECHANISM, PHARMACOKINETICS, AND DRUG INTERACTIONS:
- Buprenorphine: opioid agonist (delta and mu receptors) and antagonist (kappa receptors); naloxone: opioid antagonist.
- Metabolized primarily through CYP3A4; t ½: 24–48 hours (naloxone: 2–12 hours).
- Avoid concomitant use with opiate analgesics: diminished pain control. Additive effects with CNS depressants. CYP3A4 inhibitors and inducers may affect levels of buprenorphine.

EVIDENCE AND CLINICAL PEARLS:
- Two randomized controlled trials in adolescents and young adults, with some kids as young as 13, found buprenorphine to be safe and effective.
- C-III controlled substance. Prescribing is limited to physicians who have met qualification criteria and have received a DEA number specific to buprenorphine (see www.buprenorphine.samhsa.gov).
- Naloxone is an opioid antagonist that is active only when injected; it is added to buprenorphine in order to reduce misuse via intravenous injection of a dissolved tablet.
- The sublingual film formulation's manufacturer claims it dissolves faster and tastes better than SL tablets. Actually, it is more likely a way for the manufacturer to switch users to a "new" product (with patent protection until 2025) rather than lose patients to generics.
- SL film should be placed at base of tongue to the side of midline; this allows patient to use 2 films at the same time if dose dictates.
- Zubsolv and Bunavail formulations have better bioavailability, hence the dose equivalencies noted above.
- Prescribers should be aware of the high risk for diversion and sale of buprenorphine films and tablets. Some regular opioid abusers periodically buy buprenorphine "off the street" and use it to combat cravings and withdrawal symptoms if their drug of choice is not readily available.

FUN FACT:
The manufacturer of Suboxone, Reckitt Benckiser, generates most of its revenue from selling home and personal care products like Lysol cleaners and Durex condoms.

BOTTOM LINE:
The combination product is preferred over buprenorphine alone for maintenance because the addition of naloxone affords it a lower potential for injection abuse. Although the SL film formulation is currently priced the same as the SL tablets, the SL film strips provide very little (if any) meaningful benefits, and generic SL tablets should be used as a cost-saving measure.

DISULFIRAM (Antabuse) Fact Sheet [G]

PEDIATRIC FDA INDICATIONS:
None.

ADULT FDA INDICATIONS:
Alcohol dependence.

OFF-LABEL USES:
None.

DOSAGE FORMS:
Tablets (G): 250 mg, 500 mg.

DOSAGE GUIDANCE (ADULTS):
Start 125 mg QPM (must be abstinent from alcohol >12 hours), increase to 250 mg QPM after several days. Maintenance is usually 250 mg–500 mg QPM, but some patients can drink alcohol without a reaction at the 250 mg/day dose.

MONITORING: LFTs.

COST: $$

SIDE EFFECTS:
- Most common: skin eruptions (eg, acne, allergic dermatitis), drowsiness, fatigue, impotence, headache, metallic taste.
- Serious but rare: Severe (very rarely fatal) hepatitis or hepatic failure has been reported and may occur in patients with or without prior history of abnormal hepatic function. Rare psychotic episodes have been reported. Rarely may cause peripheral neuropathy or optic neuritis.

MECHANISM, PHARMACOKINETICS, AND DRUG INTERACTIONS:
- Aldehyde dehydrogenase inhibitor.
- Metabolized primarily through CYP450; t ½: not defined, but elimination from body is slow, and effects may persist for 1 or 2 weeks after last dose.
- While taking disulfiram, and for 1–2 weeks after stopping, avoid concomitant use of any medications containing alcohol (including topicals), metronidazole, or "disguised" forms of ethanol (cough syrup, some mouthwashes, oral solutions or liquid concentrates containing alcohol such as sertraline). Avoid vinegars, cider, extracts, and foods containing ethanol.

EVIDENCE AND CLINICAL PEARLS:
- Disulfiram has been studied and benefit has been shown in adolescents. Use in adolescents may be even riskier than in adults given adolescents' impulsivity and risk-taking behaviors, somewhat limiting disulfiram's appropriateness in this population.
- Disulfiram inhibits the enzyme aldehyde dehydrogenase; when taken with alcohol, acetaldehyde levels are increased by 5- to 10-fold, causing unpleasant symptoms that include flushing, nausea, vomiting, palpitations, chest pain, vertigo, hypotension, and (in rare instances) cardiovascular collapse and death. This is the basis for its use as aversion therapy. Common advice to patients: "You'll wish you were dead, but it likely won't kill you."
- Reaction may last from 30–60 minutes to several hours or as long as alcohol remains in the bloodstream.
- Advise patients to carry an identification card or a medical alert bracelet that states they are taking the medication and lists the symptoms of the reaction and clinician contact information.
- Duration of therapy is until the patient is fully recovered and a basis for permanent self-control has been established; maintenance therapy may be required for months or even years.

FUN FACT:
Disulfiram's antiprotozoal activity may be effective in *Giardia* and *Trichomonas* infections.

BOTTOM LINE:
Since craving is not reduced by disulfiram and any alcohol ingestion could result in a reaction, noncompliance can be common. Its use should be reserved for selective, highly motivated, and thoroughly informed patients in conjunction with supportive and psychotherapeutic treatment.

METHADONE (Methadose) Fact Sheet [G]

PEDIATRIC FDA INDICATIONS:
None.

ADULT FDA INDICATIONS:
Opioid dependence; severe pain.

OFF-LABEL USES:
None.

DOSAGE FORMS:
- **Tablets (G):** 5 mg, 10 mg, 40 mg (scored),
- **Oral solution (G):** 10 mg/5 mL, 5 mg/5 mL.
- **Oral concentrate (G):** 10 mg/mL.

DOSAGE GUIDANCE (ADULTS):
Start 15–30 mg single dose; then 5–10 mg every 2–4 hours. Adjust dose to prevent withdrawal symptoms; max 40 mg on day 1. 80–120 mg per day is a common maintenance dose for opioid dependence.

MONITORING: ECG.

COST: $

SIDE EFFECTS:
- Most common: constipation, dizziness, sedation, nausea, sweating.
- Serious but rare: May prolong the QTc interval and increase risk for torsades de pointes; caution in patients at risk for QTc prolongation; usually with doses >100 mg/day. Severe respiratory depression may occur; use extreme caution during initiation, titration, and conversion from other opiates to methadone. Respiratory depressant effects occur later and persist longer than analgesic effects, possibly contributing to cases of overdose.

MECHANISM, PHARMACOKINETICS, AND DRUG INTERACTIONS:
- Opioid agonist.
- Metabolized primarily through CYP2B6, 2C19, and 3A4 (major); inhibits CYP2D6; t ½: 8–59 hours.
- High potential for interactions. Avoid concomitant use with other potent sedatives or respiratory depressants. Use with caution in patients on medications metabolized by CYP2D6, inhibit CYP3A4, prolong the QTc interval, or promote electrolyte depletion.

EVIDENCE AND CLINICAL PEARLS:
- A few studies in adolescents. Most recently, a 12-month study of 120 adolescents found methadone treatment reduced heroin use, but treatment retention was challenging (similar to adult studies).
- C-II controlled substance; distribution of 40 mg tablets restricted to authorized opioid addiction treatment facilities.
- May only be dispensed according to the Substance Abuse and Mental Health Services Administration's (SAMHSA) Center for Substance Abuse Treatment (CSAT) guidelines. Regulations vary by area; consult regulatory agencies and/or methadone treatment facilities.
- Methadone accumulates with repeated doses; dose may need reduction after 3–5 days to prevent CNS depressant effects.

FUN FACT:
A persistent but untrue urban legend claims the name "Dolophine" was coined in tribute to Adolf Hitler by its German creators. The name was in fact created after the war by the American branch of Eli Lilly, and the pejorative term "adolphine" (never an actual name of the drug) didn't appear in the US until the early 1970s.

BOTTOM LINE:
Opiate replacement therapy via methadone reduces or eliminates illicit use of opiates and criminality associated with opiate use, supporting health and social functioning. It is a harm reduction model reducing transmission of infectious diseases such as hepatitis and HIV. Disadvantages include potential for accumulation with repeated doses (which may result in toxicity), interindividual variability in pharmacokinetic parameters, potential for drug interactions, challenges associated with dose titration, stigma associated with opiate replacement therapy, and limited availability of treatment programs (nonexistent in some geographic areas, long wait lists in other areas). Methadone has long been established as an effective treatment of opioid addiction in adults, although federal regulations prohibit most methadone programs from admitting patients younger than 18 years.

NALOXONE (Evzio, Narcan Nasal Spray) Fact Sheet [G]

PEDIATRIC FDA INDICATIONS:
Emergency treatment of known or suspected opioid overdose.

ADULT FDA INDICATIONS:
Emergency treatment of known or suspected opioid overdose.

OFF-LABEL USES:
None.

DOSAGE FORMS:
- **Pre-filled auto-injector (Evzio):** 2 mg/0.4 mL.
- **Intranasal (Narcan Nasal Spray):** 2 mg/0.1 mL, 4 mg/0.1 mL.
- Generic intranasal kit may be assembled using 2 mg/2 mL prefilled needleless syringe and a mucosal atomization device nasal adapter (requires assembly at time of administration).

PEDIATRIC DOSAGE GUIDANCE:
- IV/IM/SC: Infants and children ≤5 years or ≤20 kg: 0.1 mg/kg/dose; repeat every 2–3 minutes if needed; may need to repeat doses every 20–60 minutes.
- IV/IM/SC: Children >5 years or >20 kg and adolescents: 2 mg/dose; if no response, repeat every 2–3 minutes; may need to repeat doses every 20–60 minutes.
- Intranasal: 4 mg x1, repeat every 2–3 minutes. Bystander to spray in one nostril; may repeat into other nostril with additional doses every 2–3 minutes if no or minimal response and until emergency response arrives.
- Auto-injector (adult): Bystander to administer 2 mg IM into thigh, through clothing if necessary as directed by voice prompt; may repeat with additional doses every 2–3 minutes if no or minimal response and until emergency response arrives.

MONITORING: No specific monitoring of note.

COST: auto-injector: $$$$$; intranasal: $$$; generic kit: $

SIDE EFFECTS:
Most common: symptoms of opioid withdrawal, including body aches, fever, sweating, runny nose, sneezing, piloerection, yawning, weakness, shivering or trembling, nervousness, restlessness or irritability, diarrhea, nausea or vomiting, abdominal cramps, increased blood pressure, and tachycardia.

MECHANISM, PHARMACOKINETICS, AND DRUG INTERACTIONS:
- Opioid antagonist.
- Metabolized primarily by conjugation (non-P450) in the liver; t ½: 1.36 hours.

EVIDENCE AND CLINICAL PEARLS:
- No studies specifically in kids or adolescents, but clinical use in opioid overdose situations is the same as in adults.
- Because treatment of overdose with this opioid antagonist must be performed by someone other than the patient, instruct the prescription recipient to inform local acquaintances about having naloxone rescue and ensure that they have been instructed in recognition of overdose symptoms and naloxone administration.
- Evzio comes with printed instructions on the device label as well as electronic voice instructions (there is a speaker that provides instructions to guide the user through each step of the injection).
- Most opioids have a longer duration of action than naloxone, so it's likely that overdose symptoms (CNS depression and respiratory depression) will return after initial improvement. Therefore, patients should continue to be monitored and should receive medical attention after provision of emergency dose(s).
- Intranasal forms of naloxone rescue administration, if broadly distributed to those at risk, could make overdose rescue a more acceptable and widespread practice.
- Check out the Prescribe to Prevent website (prescribetoprevent.org) for prescriber resources such as webinars, toolkits, patient education materials, and medical-legal resources. This website also provides guidance to physicians on writing a prescription for naloxone.

FUN FACT:
Naloxone was first approved for opioid overdose treatment in 1971 and is available as a very inexpensive injectable generic. These newer formulations will come at a much higher price because of the way they are formulated, making them easier to use by non-emergency provider bystanders.

BOTTOM LINE:
Naloxone rescue saves lives. Prescribe it.

NALTREXONE (ReVia, Vivitrol) Fact Sheet [G]

PEDIATRIC FDA INDICATIONS:
None.

ADULT FDA INDICATIONS:
Alcohol dependence; opioid addiction (relapse prevention following detox).

OFF-LABEL USES:
Self-injurious behavior, irritability in autism spectrum disorder.

DOSAGE FORMS:
- **Tablets (ReVia, G):** 50 mg (scored).
- **Long-acting injection (Vivitrol):** 380 mg.

DOSAGE GUIDANCE (ADULTS):
- Opioid dependence: Start 25 mg for 1 day; if no withdrawal signs, increase to and maintain 50 mg/day (with food); doses >50 mg may increase risk of hepatoxicity.
- Alcohol dependence: Start and maintain 50 mg QD.
- Injection: 380 mg IM (gluteal) Q4 weeks (for opioid or alcohol dependence). Do not initiate therapy until patient is opioid-free for at least 7–10 days (by urinalysis).

MONITORING: LFTs.

COST: tablet: $; injection: $$$$$

SIDE EFFECTS:
- Most common: headache, nausea, somnolence, vomiting.
- Serious but rare: black box warning: dose-related hepatocellular injury, with a narrow therapeutic window, about ≤5-fold safe vs hepatotoxic. Discontinue if signs/symptoms of acute hepatitis develop.

MECHANISM, PHARMACOKINETICS, AND DRUG INTERACTIONS:
- Opioid antagonist. No significant interactions other than avoiding use with opiates (see below).
- Metabolized primarily through non-CYP450 pathway; t ½: 4 hours (5–10 days for IM).

EVIDENCE AND CLINICAL PEARLS:
- Efficacy (oral) in adults with alcohol dependence (craving and relapse) is more convincing than in opiate dependence, where craving is not decreased but euphoric effects are blocked. Monthly IM may be more effective than oral at maintaining abstinence in opiate dependence (better medication adherence).
- Naltrexone in adolescents has 2 very small studies in which it was found to reduce craving and alcohol use.
- May precipitate acute withdrawal (pain, hypertension, sweating, agitation, and irritability) in opiate-using patients; ensure patient is opioid-free for at least 7–10 days prior to initiating.
- In naltrexone-treated patients requiring emergency pain management, consider alternatives to opiates (eg, regional analgesia, non-opioid analgesics, general anesthesia). If opioid therapy is required, patients should be under the direct care of a trained anesthesia provider.
- In addition to the 25–50 mg doses, smaller compounded amounts of 3–5 mg, called low-dose naltrexone (LDN), are often used for irritability in ASD.

FUN FACT:
Methylnaltrexone, a closely related drug, is marketed as Relistor for the treatment of opioid-induced constipation.

BOTTOM LINE:
Naltrexone is used for alcohol dependence more than for opiate dependence, to minimize severity of drinking, while acamprosate is used to prevent relapse. Avoid it in patients with hepatic impairment or those taking opiate medications. For opioid dependence, methadone and buprenorphine are more effective, although naltrexone may be appropriate for highly motivated opiate-dependent patients, with injectable preferred over oral.

NICOTINE GUM/LOZENGE (Nicorette) Fact Sheet [G]

PEDIATRIC FDA INDICATIONS:
None.

ADULT FDA INDICATIONS:
Smoking cessation.

OFF-LABEL USES:
None.

DOSAGE FORMS:
- **Gum (G):** 2 mg, 4 mg (over the counter).
- **Lozenges (G):** 2 mg, 4 mg (over the counter).

DOSAGE GUIDANCE (ADULTS):
- Chew 1 piece of gum PRN urge to smoke, up to 24 pieces/day. Patients who smoke <25 cigarettes/day should start with 2 mg strength; patients smoking ≥25 cigarettes/day should start with the 4 mg strength. Use the following 12-week dosing schedule: weeks 1–6: chew 1 piece of gum every 1–2 hours; to increase chances of quitting, chew at least 9 pieces/day during the first 6 weeks; weeks 7–9: chew 1 piece of gum every 2–4 hours; weeks 10–12: chew 1 piece of gum every 4–8 hours.
- For lozenges: Patients who smoke their first cigarette within 30 minutes of waking should use 4 mg strength; otherwise 2 mg strength is recommended. Use the following 12-week dosing schedule: weeks 1–6: 1 lozenge every 1–2 hours; weeks 7–9: 1 lozenge every 2–4 hours; weeks 10–12: 1 lozenge every 4–8 hours. Use at least 9 lozenges/day during first 6 weeks to improve chances of quitting; do not use more than 1 lozenge at a time; maximum is 5 lozenges every 6 hours or 20 lozenges/day.
- Patients should be advised to completely stop smoking upon initiation of therapy.

MONITORING: No specific monitoring of note.

COST: $

SIDE EFFECTS:
Most common: headache; indigestion; nausea; hiccups; tongue, mouth, and throat irritation or tingling; jaw ache (gum).

MECHANISM, PHARMACOKINETICS, AND DRUG INTERACTIONS:
- Nicotinic-cholinergic receptor agonist.
- Metabolized primarily through liver as well as kidneys and lungs; t ½: 1–2 hours.
- Minimal risk for drug interactions. Successful cessation of smoking may increase serum levels of medications metabolized by CYP1A2 (eg, clozapine, olanzapine, theophylline), which is induced by hydrocarbons in smoke; nicotine itself has no effect.

EVIDENCE AND CLINICAL PEARLS:
- One study in adolescents showed somewhat higher compliance with patch therapy than with gum, but this may vary with patient preference.
- If there are cravings throughout the day even with a patch, add a short-acting agent (gum, lozenge, spray, inhaler). Discuss chewing technique for gum: Chew a few times (about 15 times) to activate the release (the sign is tingling/bad peppery taste), then park between cheek and gum until tingle is gone (about 1 minute), and switch sides every few minutes. Repeat until most of the tingle is gone (~30 minutes). Each piece is 2 mg or 4 mg and lasts about 30 minutes.
- Lozenges should not be chewed or swallowed; allow to dissolve slowly (~20–30 minutes).
- Heavy smokers should use higher-dose gum or lozenge and at least 9 pieces/day to maximize chances of success. Do not use more than 1 piece at a time.
- Each 4 mg lozenge or gum results in 2 mg of absorbed nicotine, equivalent to 2 cigarettes.

FUN FACT:
Nicotine gum is available in a variety of flavors: fruit, mint, cinnamon, orange, cherry, and "original."

BOTTOM LINE:
First-line intervention for those patients who can stop smoking at initiation of therapy; nicotine in the form of gum or lozenge may act as a substitute oral activity, which may aid in behavior modification.

NICOTINE INHALED (Nicotrol Inhaler) Fact Sheet

PEDIATRIC FDA INDICATIONS:
None.

ADULT FDA INDICATIONS:
Smoking cessation.

OFF-LABEL USES:
None.

DOSAGE FORMS:
Cartridges: 4 mg delivered per 10 mg cartridge (prescription required).

DOSAGE GUIDANCE (ADULTS):
- Use frequent continuous puffing for 20 minutes with each cartridge; 80 deep inhalations over 20 minutes releases 4 mg nicotine, of which 2 mg is absorbed. Use 6–16 cartridges per day. Taper after 6–12 weeks of use by gradual dose reduction over 6–12 additional weeks.
- Patients should be advised to completely stop smoking upon initiation of therapy.

MONITORING: No specific monitoring of note.

COST: $$$$

SIDE EFFECTS:
Most common: headache, mouth/throat irritation, dyspepsia, cough, unpleasant taste, rhinitis, tearing, sneezing.

MECHANISM, PHARMACOKINETICS, AND DRUG INTERACTIONS:
- Nicotinic-cholinergic receptor agonist.
- Metabolized primarily through liver as well as kidneys and lungs; t ½: 1–2 hours.
- Minimal drug interactions. Successful cessation of smoking may increase serum levels of medications metabolized by CYP1A2 (eg, clozapine, olanzapine, theophylline), which is induced by hydrocarbons in smoke; nicotine itself has no effect.

EVIDENCE AND CLINICAL PEARLS:
- No data specifically in kids or adolescents.
- Insert cartridge into inhaler and push hard until it pops into place. Replace mouthpiece and twist the top and bottom so that markings do not line up. Inhale deeply into the back of the throat or puff in short breaths. Nicotine in cartridge is used up after about 20 minutes of active puffing.
- Do not eat or drink 15 minutes before or during use. Puffing lightly rather than inhaling reduces coughing.
- Irritation in the mouth and throat may occur in about 40% of patients; coughing (32%) and rhinitis (23%) are also common. These effects are generally mild and abate with continued use. Use with caution in patients with bronchospastic disease due to potential airway irritation (consider other forms of nicotine replacement).
- Higher ambient temperatures deliver more nicotine; lower temperatures deliver less.
- 1 cartridge delivers 80 puffs or about 2 mg of absorbed nicotine. Roughly 10 cartridges per day is equivalent to the nicotine of smoking 1 pack per day.

FUN FACT:
A nicotine inhaler is not really a true inhaler; puffing deposits the nicotine into the mouth, and it is then absorbed in the same manner as the nicotine gum or lozenge preparations.

BOTTOM LINE:
Very high expense and unpleasant side effects make this form of nicotine replacement therapy difficult to recommend as a first-line option since no single therapy has been shown to be more effective than another.

NICOTINE NASAL SPRAY (Nicotrol NS) Fact Sheet

PEDIATRIC FDA INDICATIONS:
None.

ADULT FDA INDICATIONS:
Smoking cessation.

OFF-LABEL USES:
None.

DOSAGE FORMS:
10 mL bottle: 10 mg/mL delivering 0.5 mg/spray in 200 sprays (prescription required).

DOSAGE GUIDANCE (ADULTS):
- Use 1–2 sprays/hour as needed; do not exceed more than 5 doses (10 sprays) per hour. Max dose is 40 doses/day (80 sprays). Each dose (2 sprays) contains 1 mg of nicotine.
- After initial 8 weeks of treatment, taper dose gradually over 4–6 weeks.
- Patients should be advised to completely stop smoking upon initiation of therapy.

MONITORING: No specific monitoring of note.

COST: $$$$

SIDE EFFECTS:
Most common: headache, dyspepsia, rhinitis, nasal irritation, sneezing, coughing.

MECHANISM, PHARMACOKINETICS, AND DRUG INTERACTIONS:
- Nicotinic-cholinergic receptor agonist.
- Metabolized primarily through liver as well as kidneys and lungs; t ½: 1–2 hours.
- Minimal risk for drug interactions. Successful cessation of smoking may increase serum levels of medications metabolized by CYP1A2 (eg, clozapine, olanzapine, theophylline), which is induced by hydrocarbons in smoke; nicotine itself has no effect.

EVIDENCE AND CLINICAL PEARLS:
- Nicotine nasal spray was not well-tolerated in a randomized open-label trial with 40 adolescent smokers. More than half (57%) dropped out of the study after only a week. The most common complaints were nasal irritation and burning, and complaints about the taste and smell.
- Prime pump prior to first use. Blow nose gently prior to use. Tilt head back slightly, breathe through mouth, and spray once in each nostril. Do not sniff, swallow, or inhale through nose.
- Moderate to severe nasal irritation in 94% of patients in the first 2 days of use; severity decreases over time. Nasal congestion and transient changes in sense of smell and taste also reported. Avoid in patients with chronic nasal disorders (eg, allergy, rhinitis, nasal polyps, and sinusitis). Exacerbations of bronchospasm reported in patients with asthma.
- Heavy smokers may well use the maximum amount of 80 sprays/day, meaning they would need a new bottle every 2–3 days. This can be tremendously and prohibitively expensive.
- Potential for abuse and dependence appears to be greater than with other NRT.

FUN FACT:
In a published case report (*Am J Psychiatry* 2001), a 54-year-old man who could no longer afford his Nicotrol NS prescription found a commercial source for nicotine on the Internet (sold as an insecticide). He purchased 25 g in a 1 g/mL solution for $30, diluted the nicotine solution with distilled water to 10 mg/mL, and then placed the solution into empty spray bottles.

BOTTOM LINE:
The idea of nasal administration of nicotine is appealing in that it more closely approximates the time course of plasma nicotine levels observed after cigarette smoking than other dosage forms; however, the high cost coupled with unpleasant side effects make this difficult to recommend as a first-line treatment, especially since no one form of nicotine replacement therapy has been shown to be more effective than another.

NICOTINE PATCH (Nicoderm CQ) Fact Sheet [G]

PEDIATRIC FDA INDICATIONS:
None.

ADULT FDA INDICATIONS:
Smoking cessation.

OFF-LABEL USES:
None.

DOSAGE FORMS:
Transdermal patch (G): 7 mg, 14 mg, 21 mg/24 hours (over the counter).

DOSAGE GUIDANCE (ADULTS):
- Apply new patch every 24 hours (same time each day, usually after awakening) to non-hairy, clean, dry skin on the upper body or upper outer arm; each patch should be applied to a different site. Adjustment may be required during initial treatment (increase dose if experiencing withdrawal symptoms; lower dose if experiencing side effects). Patients smoking >10 cigarettes/day: Start with 21 mg/day for 6 weeks, then 14 mg/day for 2 weeks, then 7 mg/day for 2 weeks. Patients smoking ≤10 cigarettes/day: Start with 14 mg/day for 6 weeks, then 7 mg/day for 2 weeks.
- Patients should be advised to completely stop smoking upon initiation of therapy.

MONITORING: No specific monitoring of note.

COST: $

SIDE EFFECTS:
Most common: application site reactions (itching, burning, or redness), diarrhea, dyspepsia, abdominal pain.

MECHANISM, PHARMACOKINETICS, AND DRUG INTERACTIONS:
- Nicotinic-cholinergic receptor agonist.
- Metabolized primarily through liver as well as kidneys and lungs; t ½: 3–6 hours.
- Minimal risk for drug interactions. Successful cessation of smoking may increase serum levels of medications metabolized by CYP1A2 (eg, clozapine, olanzapine, theophylline), which is induced by hydrocarbons in smoke; nicotine itself has no effect.

EVIDENCE AND CLINICAL PEARLS:
- Nicotine patch therapy has been shown to be safe and effective for smoking cessation in adolescent smokers.
- One study in adolescents showed somewhat higher compliance with patch than with gum, but this may vary with patient preference.
- Start most patients who want to quit smoking on NRT. Prescribe patch based on nicotine load: 1 ppd = 21 mg patch. Place it at the same time each day, usually in the morning. Start above the heart and rotate left around the body to prevent skin irritation. Use 0.5% cortisone cream for irritation/rash. Initial dose for 4–8 weeks, then taper monthly or every 2 months. Advise no smoking—patients may note nausea or racing heart if they do.
- Patch may be worn for 16 or 24 hours. If craving upon awakening, wear patch for 24 hours; if vivid dreams or sleep disruptions occur, wear patch for 16 hours, then remove at bedtime.
- Do not cut patch; this causes rapid evaporation, making the patch useless.
- Up to 50% of patients will experience a local skin reaction, which is usually mild and self-limiting but may worsen with continued treatment. Local treatment with hydrocortisone cream 1% or triamcinolone cream 0.5% and rotating patch sites may help. In fewer than 5% of patients, such reactions require discontinuation.

FUN FACTS:
- In the U.S., nicotine patches and gum are available by prescription only for patients under 18 years (they are available over the counter for adults).
- In a particularly ironic scene in the dark comedy *Thank You for Smoking*, nicotine patches are used by antismoking "terrorists" to try to harm a marketing executive for Big Tobacco. The attempt fails because the executive already has a very high tolerance to nicotine, resulting in the headline "Smoking Saved My Life."

BOTTOM LINE:
Nicotine patches are a first-line intervention in patients who are able to quit smoking at initiation of treatment and who are regular and constant smokers.

VARENICLINE (Chantix) Fact Sheet

PEDIATRIC FDA INDICATIONS:
None.

ADULT FDA INDICATIONS:
Smoking cessation.

OFF-LABEL USES:
None.

DOSAGE FORMS:
Tablets: 0.5 mg, 1 mg.

DOSAGE GUIDANCE (ADULTS):
Start 0.5 mg QD x 3 days, ↑ to 0.5 mg BID x 4 days then ↑ to 1 mg BID for 11 weeks. Titrate slowly and take with food and a full glass of water to decrease GI upset. Start 1 week before target quit date; may consider setting a quit date up to 35 days after starting varenicline (to improve likelihood of abstinence).

MONITORING: No specific monitoring of note.

COST: $$$$

SIDE EFFECTS:
- Most common: nausea, insomnia, headache, abnormal dreams, constipation, flatulence.
- Serious but rare: neuropsychiatric events (eg, depression, suicidal thoughts, suicide, psychosis, hostility) reported, even without preexisting psychiatric disease. Warning recently revised as risk is lower than previously thought.

MECHANISM, PHARMACOKINETICS, AND DRUG INTERACTIONS:
- Nicotine receptor partial agonist.
- Excreted mostly unchanged with minimal hepatic (non-CYP450) metabolism; t ½: 24 hours.
- Potential lowered tolerance to alcohol, with psychiatric reactions. H2 blockers, quinolones, and trimethoprim may increase varenicline levels. Smoking cessation may alter pharmacokinetics of clozapine, olanzapine, theophylline, warfarin, insulin, and others.

EVIDENCE AND CLINICAL PEARLS:
- An 8-week randomized double-blind pilot in 29 smokers aged 15–20 found higher rates of smoking cessation and greater reduction in number of cigarettes per day with varenicline than bupropion, but the trial was not adequately powered for comparison.
- Dual mechanism: partial agonist, mimicking nicotine effects on the brain and reducing withdrawal; also blocks nicotine binding, decreasing the reinforcing effect of smoking.
- If patient successfully quits smoking after 12 weeks, continue for another 12 weeks. If not successful in first 12 weeks, then discontinue and reassess factors contributing to failure.
- Similar quit rates as bupropion at 6 months (25%), but higher quit rates compared to bupropion at 1 year if a second 12-week course of varenicline is used.
- Can be combined with bupropion; use with nicotine replacement therapies likely to lead to increased side effects, particularly nausea, headache, vomiting, and dizziness.
- Recently touted for use in autism. Several case reports of improvement, but no other research exists.
- Discuss insomnia and vivid dreams with patients. Psychiatric side effects (eg, depression, suicidal ideation, and aggression) are likely caused by nicotine withdrawal, not Chantix.

FUN FACT:
The show *Saturday Night Live* aired a parody of a Chantix commercial suggesting that the side effects of *quitting* smoking could be dangerous (it's on YouTube).

BOTTOM LINE:
Varenicline is the most effective tobacco cessation medication in adults but lacks data in adolescents, safety concerns aside. Psychiatric side effects are usually limited to insomnia or abnormal dreams. Dramatic reactions are possible but rare.

Appendices

APPENDIX A: BLOOD PRESSURE PARAMETERS FOR CHILDREN

Blood Pressure Levels for Boys by Age and Height Percentile

Age (Year)	BP Percentile ↓	Systolic BP (mmHg) ← Percentile of Height →							Diastolic BP (mmHg) ← Percentile of Height →						
		5th	10th	25th	50th	75th	90th	95th	5th	10th	25th	50th	75th	90th	95th
1	50th	80	81	83	85	87	88	89	34	35	36	37	38	39	39
	90th	94	95	97	99	100	102	103	49	50	51	52	53	53	54
	95th	98	99	101	103	104	106	106	54	54	55	56	57	58	58
	99th	105	106	108	110	112	113	114	61	62	63	64	65	66	66
2	50th	84	85	87	88	90	92	92	39	40	41	42	43	44	44
	90th	97	99	100	102	104	105	106	54	55	56	57	58	58	59
	95th	101	102	104	106	108	109	110	59	59	60	61	62	63	63
	99th	109	110	111	113	115	117	117	66	67	68	69	70	71	71
3	50th	86	87	89	91	93	94	95	44	44	45	46	47	48	48
	90th	100	101	103	105	107	108	109	59	59	60	61	62	63	63
	95th	104	105	107	109	110	112	113	63	63	64	65	66	67	67
	99th	111	112	114	116	118	119	120	71	71	72	73	74	75	75
4	50th	88	89	91	93	95	96	97	47	48	49	50	51	51	52
	90th	102	103	105	107	109	110	111	62	63	64	65	66	66	67
	95th	106	107	109	111	112	114	115	66	67	68	69	70	71	71
	99th	113	114	116	118	120	121	122	74	75	76	77	78	78	79
5	50th	90	91	93	95	96	98	98	50	51	52	53	54	55	55
	90th	104	105	106	108	110	111	112	65	66	67	68	69	69	70
	95th	108	109	110	112	114	115	116	69	70	71	72	73	74	74
	99th	115	116	118	120	121	123	123	77	78	79	80	81	81	82
6	50th	91	92	94	96	98	99	100	53	53	54	55	56	57	57
	90th	105	106	108	110	111	113	113	68	68	69	70	71	72	72
	95th	109	110	112	114	115	117	117	72	72	73	74	75	76	76
	99th	116	117	119	121	123	124	125	80	80	81	82	83	84	84
7	50th	92	94	95	97	99	100	101	55	55	56	57	58	59	59
	90th	106	107	109	111	113	114	115	70	70	71	72	73	74	74
	95th	110	111	113	115	117	118	119	74	74	75	76	77	78	78
	99th	117	118	120	122	124	125	126	82	82	83	84	85	86	86
8	50th	94	95	97	99	100	102	102	56	57	58	59	60	60	61
	90th	107	109	110	112	114	115	116	71	72	72	73	74	75	76
	95th	111	112	114	116	118	119	120	75	76	77	78	79	79	80
	99th	119	120	122	123	125	127	127	83	84	85	86	87	87	88
9	50th	95	96	98	100	102	103	104	57	58	59	60	61	61	62
	90th	109	110	112	114	115	117	118	72	73	74	75	76	76	77
	95th	113	114	116	118	119	121	121	76	77	78	79	80	81	81
	99th	120	121	123	125	127	128	129	84	85	86	87	88	88	89
10	50th	97	98	100	102	103	105	106	58	59	60	61	61	62	63
	90th	111	112	114	115	117	119	119	73	73	74	75	76	77	78
	95th	115	116	117	119	121	122	123	77	78	79	80	81	81	82
	99th	122	123	125	127	128	130	130	85	86	86	88	88	89	90

Source: https://www.nhlbi.nih.gov

Blood Pressure Levels for Boys by Age and Height Percentile (Continued)

Age (Year)	BP Percentile ↓	Systolic BP (mmHg) ← Percentile of Height →							Diastolic BP (mmHg) ← Percentile of Height →						
		5th	10th	25th	50th	75th	90th	95th	5th	10th	25th	50th	75th	90th	95th
11	50th	99	100	102	104	105	107	107	59	59	60	61	62	63	63
	90th	113	114	115	117	119	120	121	74	74	75	76	77	78	78
	95th	117	118	119	121	123	124	125	78	78	79	80	81	82	82
	99th	124	125	127	129	130	132	132	86	86	87	88	89	90	90
12	50th	101	102	104	106	108	109	110	59	60	61	62	63	63	64
	90th	115	116	118	120	121	123	123	74	75	75	76	77	78	79
	95th	119	120	122	123	125	127	127	78	79	80	81	82	82	83
	99th	126	127	129	131	133	134	135	86	87	88	89	90	90	91
13	50th	104	105	106	108	110	111	112	60	60	61	62	63	64	64
	90th	117	118	120	122	124	125	126	75	75	76	77	78	79	79
	95th	121	122	124	126	128	129	130	79	79	80	81	82	83	83
	99th	128	130	131	133	135	136	137	87	87	88	89	90	91	91
14	50th	106	107	109	111	113	114	115	60	61	62	63	64	65	65
	90th	120	121	123	125	126	128	128	75	76	77	78	79	79	80
	95th	124	125	127	128	130	132	132	80	80	81	82	83	84	84
	99th	131	132	134	136	138	139	140	87	88	89	90	91	92	92
15	50th	109	110	112	113	115	117	117	61	62	63	64	65	66	66
	90th	122	124	125	127	129	130	131	76	77	78	79	80	80	81
	95th	126	127	129	131	133	134	135	81	81	82	83	84	85	85
	99th	134	135	136	138	140	142	142	88	89	90	91	92	93	93
16	50th	111	112	114	116	118	119	120	63	63	64	65	66	67	67
	90th	125	126	128	130	131	133	134	78	78	79	80	81	82	82
	95th	129	130	132	134	135	137	137	82	83	83	84	85	86	87
	99th	136	137	139	141	143	144	145	90	90	91	92	93	94	94
17	50th	114	115	116	118	120	121	122	65	66	66	67	68	69	70
	90th	127	128	130	132	134	135	136	80	80	81	82	83	84	84
	95th	131	132	134	136	138	139	140	84	85	86	87	87	88	89
	99th	139	140	141	143	145	146	147	92	93	93	94	95	96	97

BP, blood pressure

* The 90th percentile is 1.28 SD, 95th percentile is 1.645 SD, and the 99th percentile is 2.326 SD over the mean.

For research purposes, the standard deviations in Appendix Table B–1 allow one to compute BP Z-scores and percentiles for boys with height percentiles given in Table 3 (i.e., the 5th, 10th, 25th, 50th, 75th, 90th, and 95th percentiles). These height percentiles must be converted to height Z-scores given by (5% = -1.645; 10% = -1.28; 25% = -0.68; 50% = 0; 75% = 0.68; 90% = 1.28%; 95% = 1.645) and then computed according to the methodology in steps 2–4 described in Appendix B. For children with height percentiles other than these, follow steps 1–4 as described in Appendix B.

Source: https://www.nhlbi.nih.gov

Blood Pressure Levels for Girls by Age and Height Percentile

Age (Year)	BP Percentile ↓	Systolic BP (mmHg) ← Percentile of Height →							Diastolic BP (mmHg) ← Percentile of Height →						
		5th	10th	25th	50th	75th	90th	95th	5th	10th	25th	50th	75th	90th	95th
1	50th	83	84	85	86	88	89	90	38	39	39	40	41	41	42
	90th	97	97	98	100	101	102	103	52	53	53	54	55	55	56
	95th	100	101	102	104	105	106	107	56	57	57	58	59	59	60
	99th	108	108	109	111	112	113	114	64	64	65	65	66	67	67
2	50th	85	85	87	88	89	91	91	43	44	44	45	46	46	47
	90th	98	99	100	101	103	104	105	57	58	58	59	60	61	61
	95th	102	103	104	105	107	108	109	61	62	62	63	64	65	65
	99th	109	110	111	112	114	115	116	69	69	70	70	71	72	72
3	50th	86	87	88	89	91	92	93	47	48	48	49	50	50	51
	90th	100	100	102	103	104	106	106	61	62	62	63	64	64	65
	95th	104	104	105	107	108	109	110	65	66	66	67	68	68	69
	99th	111	111	113	114	115	116	117	73	73	74	74	75	76	76
4	50th	88	88	90	91	92	94	94	50	50	51	52	52	53	54
	90th	101	102	103	104	106	107	108	64	64	65	66	67	67	68
	95th	105	106	107	108	110	111	112	68	68	69	70	71	71	72
	99th	112	113	114	115	117	118	119	76	76	76	77	78	79	79
5	50th	89	90	91	93	94	95	96	52	53	53	54	55	55	56
	90th	103	103	105	106	107	109	109	66	67	67	68	69	69	70
	95th	107	107	108	110	111	112	113	70	71	71	72	73	73	74
	99th	114	114	116	117	118	120	120	78	78	79	79	80	81	81
6	50th	91	92	93	94	96	97	98	54	54	55	56	56	57	58
	90th	104	105	106	108	109	110	111	68	68	69	70	70	71	72
	95th	108	109	110	111	113	114	115	72	72	73	74	74	75	76
	99th	115	116	117	119	120	121	122	80	80	80	81	82	83	83
7	50th	93	93	95	96	97	99	99	55	56	56	57	58	58	59
	90th	106	107	108	109	111	112	113	69	70	70	71	72	72	73
	95th	110	111	112	113	115	116	116	73	74	74	75	76	76	77
	99th	117	118	119	120	122	123	124	81	81	82	82	83	84	84
8	50th	95	95	96	98	99	100	101	57	57	57	58	59	60	60
	90th	108	109	110	111	113	114	114	71	71	71	72	73	74	74
	95th	112	112	114	115	116	118	118	75	75	75	76	77	78	78
	99th	119	120	121	122	123	125	125	82	82	83	83	84	85	86
9	50th	96	97	98	100	101	102	103	58	58	58	59	60	61	61
	90th	110	110	112	113	114	116	116	72	72	72	73	74	75	75
	95th	114	114	115	117	118	119	120	76	76	76	77	78	79	79
	99th	121	121	123	124	125	127	127	83	83	84	84	85	86	87
10	50th	98	99	100	102	103	104	105	59	59	59	60	61	62	62
	90th	112	112	114	115	116	118	118	73	73	73	74	75	76	76
	95th	116	116	117	119	120	121	122	77	77	77	78	79	80	80
	99th	123	123	125	126	127	129	129	84	84	85	86	86	87	88

Source: https://www.nhlbi.nih.gov

Blood Pressure Levels for Girls by Age and Height Percentile (Continued)

Age (Year)	BP Percentile ↓	Systolic BP (mmHg) ← Percentile of Height →							Diastolic BP (mmHg) ← Percentile of Height →						
		5th	10th	25th	50th	75th	90th	95th	5th	10th	25th	50th	75th	90th	95th
11	50th	100	101	102	103	105	106	107	60	60	60	61	62	63	63
	90th	114	114	116	117	118	119	120	74	74	74	75	76	77	77
	95th	118	118	119	121	122	123	124	78	78	78	79	80	81	81
	99th	125	125	126	128	129	130	131	85	85	86	87	87	88	89
12	50th	102	103	104	105	107	108	109	61	61	61	62	63	64	64
	90th	116	116	117	119	120	121	122	75	75	75	76	77	78	78
	95th	119	120	121	123	124	125	126	79	79	79	80	81	82	82
	99th	127	127	128	130	131	132	133	86	86	87	88	88	89	90
13	50th	104	105	106	107	109	110	110	62	62	62	63	64	65	65
	90th	117	118	119	121	122	123	124	76	76	76	77	78	79	79
	95th	121	122	123	124	126	127	128	80	80	80	81	82	83	83
	99th	128	129	130	132	133	134	135	87	87	88	89	89	90	91
14	50th	106	106	107	109	110	111	112	63	63	63	64	65	66	66
	90th	119	120	121	122	124	125	125	77	77	77	78	79	80	80
	95th	123	123	125	126	127	129	129	81	81	81	82	83	84	84
	99th	130	131	132	133	135	136	136	88	88	89	90	90	91	92
15	50th	107	108	109	110	111	113	113	64	64	64	65	66	67	67
	90th	120	121	122	123	125	126	127	78	78	78	79	80	81	81
	95th	124	125	126	127	129	130	131	82	82	82	83	84	85	85
	99th	131	132	133	134	136	137	138	89	89	90	91	91	92	93
16	50th	108	108	110	111	112	114	114	64	64	65	66	66	67	68
	90th	121	122	123	124	126	127	128	78	78	79	80	81	81	82
	95th	125	126	127	128	130	131	132	82	82	83	84	85	85	86
	99th	132	133	134	135	137	138	139	90	90	90	91	92	93	93
17	50th	108	109	110	111	113	114	115	64	65	65	66	67	67	68
	90th	122	122	123	125	126	127	128	78	79	79	80	81	81	82
	95th	125	126	127	129	130	131	132	82	83	83	84	85	85	86
	99th	133	133	134	136	137	138	139	90	90	91	91	92	93	93

BP, blood pressure

* The 90th percentile is 1.28 SD, 95th percentile is 1.645 SD, and the 99th percentile is 2.326 SD over the mean.

For research purposes, the standard deviations in Appendix Table B–1 allow one to compute BP Z-scores and percentiles for girls with height percentiles given in Table 4 (i.e., the 5th, 10th, 25th, 50th, 75th, 90th, and 95th percentiles). These height percentiles must be converted to height Z-scores given by (5% = -1.645; 10% = -1.28; 25% = -0.68; 50% = 0; 75% = 0.68; 90% = 1.28%; 95% = 1.645) and then computed according to the methodology in steps 2–4 described in Appendix B. For children with height percentiles other than these, follow steps 1–4 as described in Appendix B.

Source: https://www.nhlbi.nih.gov

APPENDIX B: GROWTH AND BODY MASS INDEX CHARTS

2 to 20 years: Boys
Body mass index-for-age percentiles

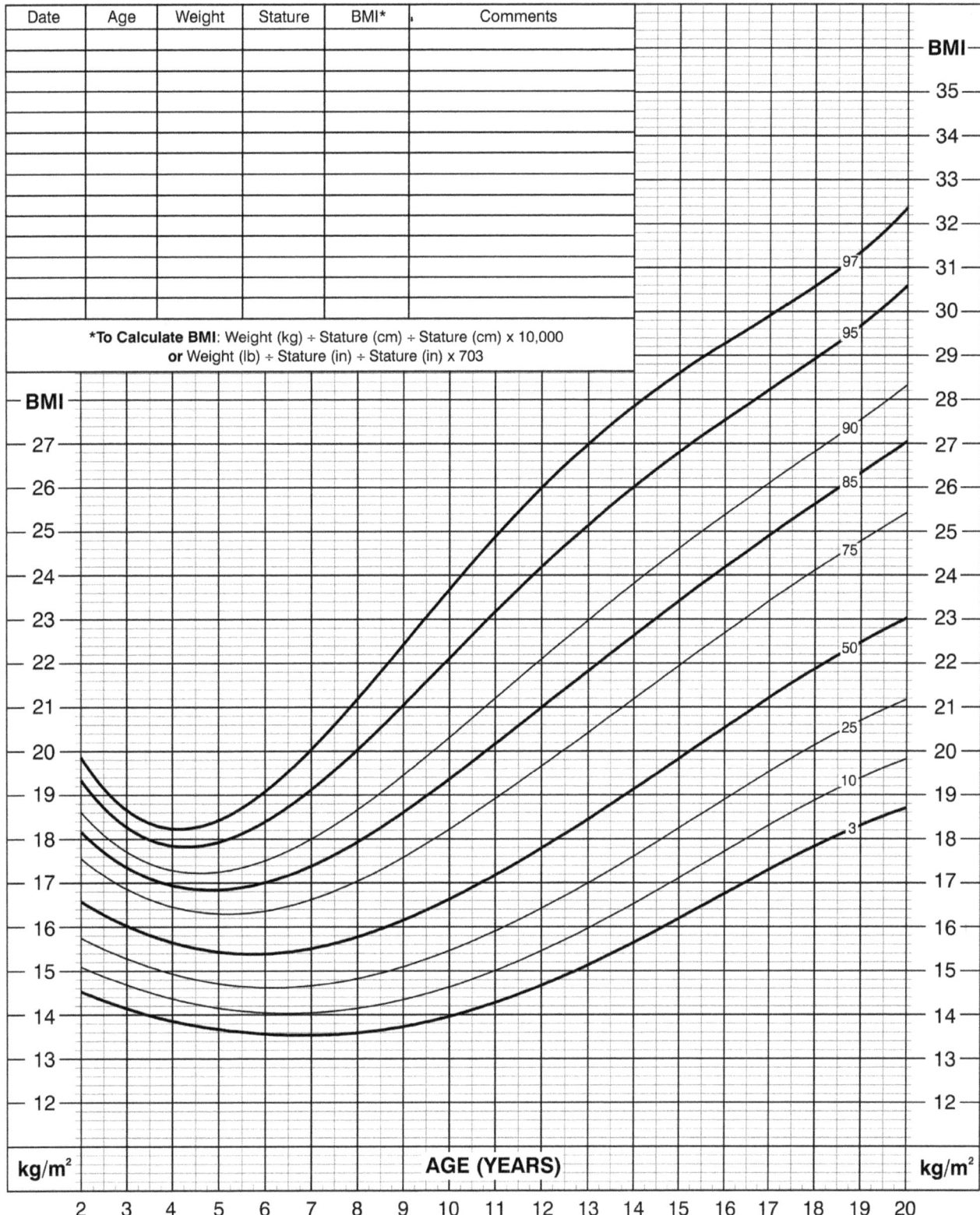

2 to 20 years: Girls
Body mass index-for-age percentiles

NAME ____________________

RECORD # ____________

Date	Age	Weight	Stature	BMI*	Comments

***To Calculate BMI**: Weight (kg) ÷ Stature (cm) ÷ Stature (cm) x 10,000
or Weight (lb) ÷ Stature (in) ÷ Stature (in) x 703

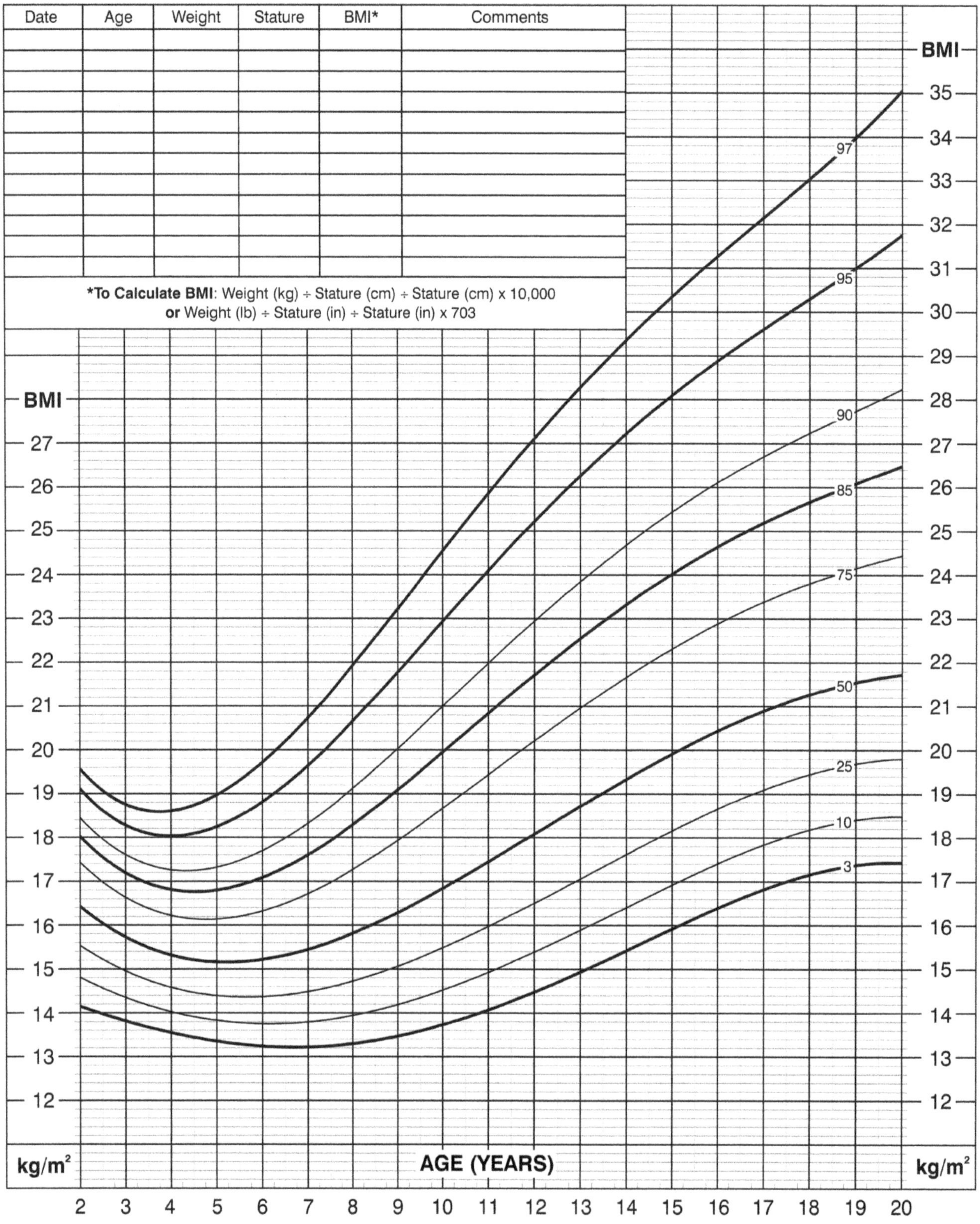

Published May 30, 2000 (modified 10/16/00).
SOURCE: Developed by the National Center for Health Statistics in collaboration with
the National Center for Chronic Disease Prevention and Health Promotion (2000).

CDC
SAFER • HEALTHIER • PEOPLE™

Source: http://www.cdc.gov/growthcharts

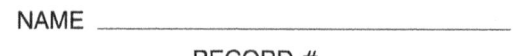

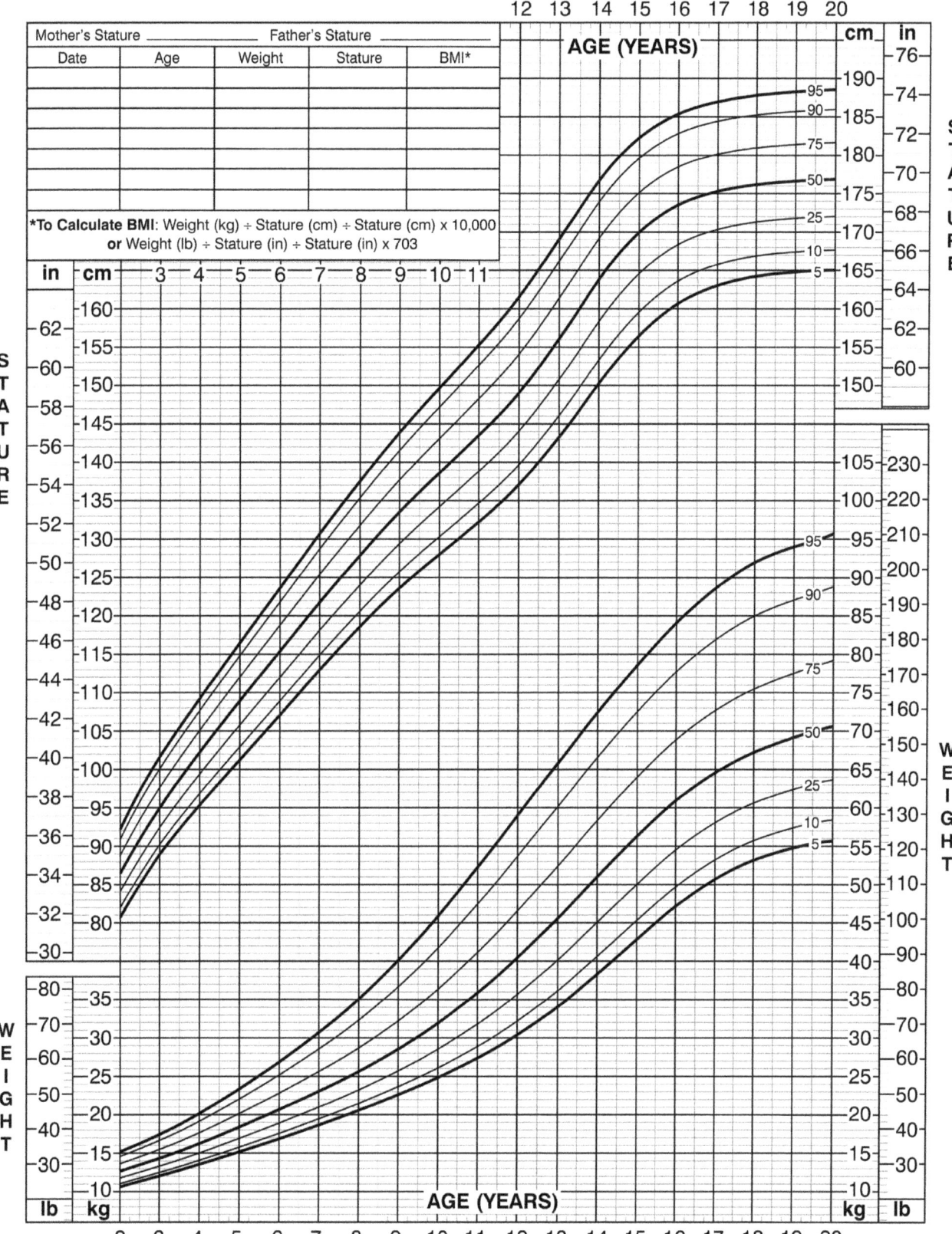

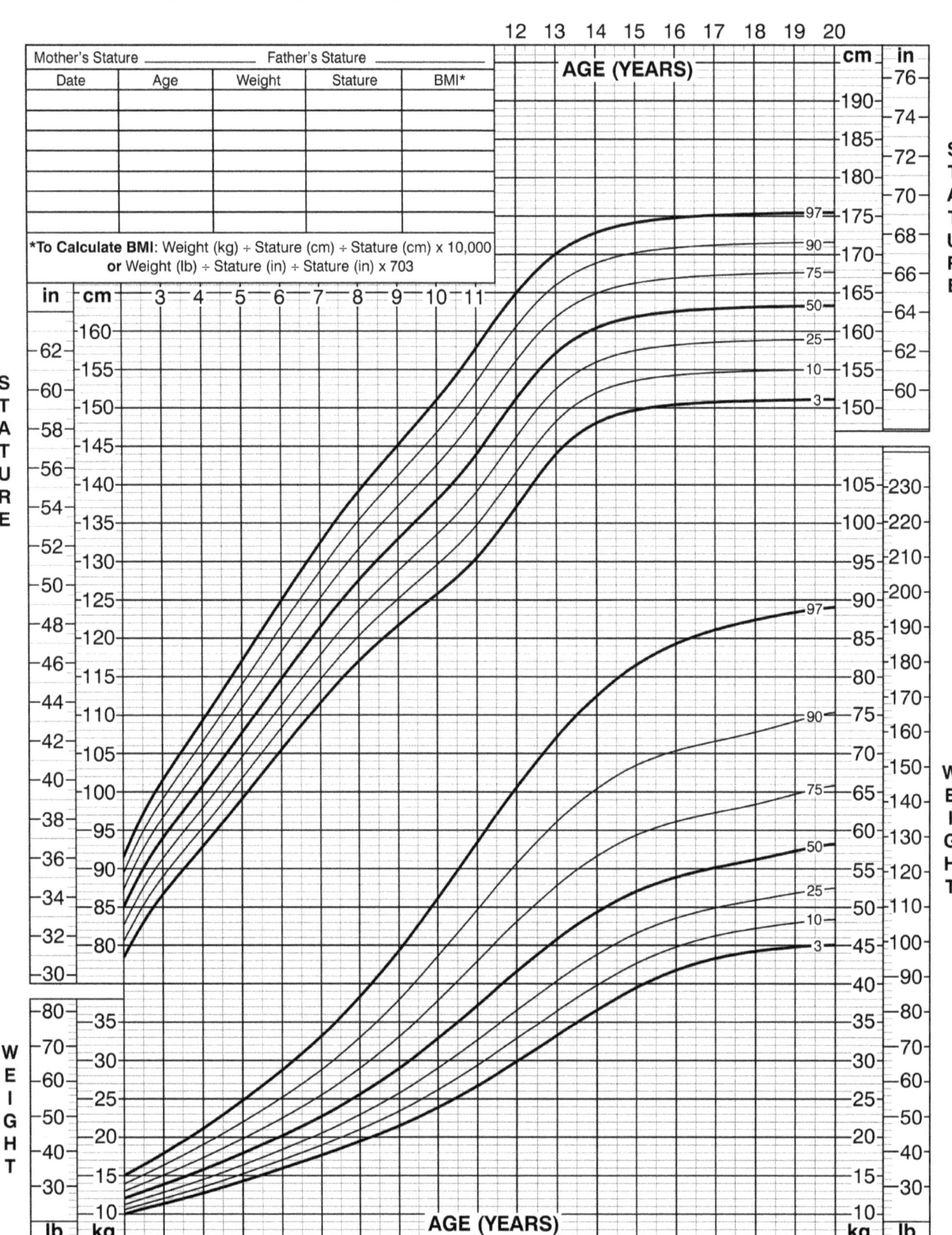

APPENDIX C: ABNORMAL INVOLUNTARY MOVEMENT SCALE (AIMS)

CODE
0=None
1=Minimal, may be extreme normal
2=Mild
3=Moderate
4=Severe

	MOVEMENT RATINGS: Rate highest severity observed. Rate movements that occur upon activation one less than those observed spontaneously. Circle movement as well as code number that applies.	RATER Date	RATER Date	RATER Date	RATER Date
Facial and Oral Movements	1. Muscles of Facial Expression eg, movements of forehead, eyebrows, periorbital area, cheeks, including frowning, blinking, smiling, grimacing	0 1 2 3 4	0 1 2 3 4	0 1 2 3 4	0 1 2 3 4
	2. Lips and Perioral Area eg, puckering, pouting, smacking	0 1 2 3 4	0 1 2 3 4	0 1 2 3 4	0 1 2 3 4
	3. Jaw eg, biting, clenching, chewing, mouth opening, lateral movement	0 1 2 3 4	0 1 2 3 4	0 1 2 3 4	0 1 2 3 4
	4. Tongue Rate only increases in movement both in and out of mouth, NOT inability to sustain movement. Darting in and out of mouth.	0 1 2 3 4	0 1 2 3 4	0 1 2 3 4	0 1 2 3 4
Extremity Movements	5. Upper (arms, wrists, hands, fingers) Include choreic movements (ie, rapid, objectively purposeless, irregular, spontaneous) athetoid movements (ie, slow, irregular, complex, serpentine). DO NOT INCLUDE TREMOR (ie, repetitive, regular, rhythmic)	0 1 2 3 4	0 1 2 3 4	0 1 2 3 4	0 1 2 3 4
	6. Lower (legs, knees, ankles, toes) eg, lateral knee movement, foot tapping, heel dropping, foot squirming, inversion and eversion of foot.	0 1 2 3 4	0 1 2 3 4	0 1 2 3 4	0 1 2 3 4
Trunk Movements	7. Neck, shoulders, hips eg, rocking, twisting, squirming, pelvic gyrations	0 1 2 3 4	0 1 2 3 4	0 1 2 3 4	0 1 2 3 4
Global Judgments	8. Severity of abnormal movements overall	0 1 2 3 4	0 1 2 3 4	0 1 2 3 4	0 1 2 3 4
	9. Incapacitation due to abnormal movements	0 1 2 3 4	0 1 2 3 4	0 1 2 3 4	0 1 2 3 4
	10. Patient's awareness of abnormal movements Rate only patient's report No awareness 0 Aware, no distress 1 Aware, mild distress 2 Aware, moderate distress 3 Aware, severe distress 4	0 1 2 3 4	0 1 2 3 4	0 1 2 3 4	0 1 2 3 4
Dental Status	11. Current problems with teeth and/or dentures?	No Yes	No Yes	No Yes	No Yes
	12. Are dentures usually worn?	No Yes	No Yes	No Yes	No Yes
	13. Edentia?	No Yes	No Yes	No Yes	No Yes
	14. Do movements disappear in sleep?	No Yes	No Yes	No Yes	No Yes

ABNORMAL INVOLUNTARY MOVEMENT SCALE (AIMS)

DEFINITION

The Abnormal Involuntary Movement Scale (AIMS) is a rating scale that was designed in the 1970s to measure involuntary movements known as tardive dyskinesia (TD). TD is a disorder that sometimes develops as a side effect of long-term treatment with neuroleptic (antipsychotic) medications.

PURPOSE

Tardive dyskinesia is a syndrome characterized by abnormal involuntary movements of the patient's face, mouth, trunk, or limbs, which affects 20%–30% of patients who have been treated for months or years with neuroleptic medications. Patients who are older, are heavy smokers, or have diabetes mellitus are at higher risk of developing TD. The movements of the patient's limbs and trunk are sometimes called choreathetoid, which means a dance-like movement that repeats itself and has no rhythm. The AIMS test is used not only to detect tardive dyskinesia but also to follow the severity of a patient's TD over time. It is a valuable tool for clinicians who are monitoring the effects of long-term treatment with neuroleptic medications and also for researchers studying the effects of these drugs. The AIMS test is given every three to six months to monitor the patient for the development of TD. For most patients, TD develops three months after the initiation of neuroleptic therapy; in elderly patients, however, TD can develop after as little as one month.

PRECAUTIONS

The AIMS test was originally developed for administration by trained clinicians. People who are not health care professionals, however, can also be taught to administer the test by completing a training seminar.

DESCRIPTION

The entire test can be completed in about 10 minutes. The AIMS test has a total of twelve items rating involuntary movements of various areas of the patient's body. These items are rated on a five-point scale of severity from 0–4. The scale is rated from 0 (none), 1 (minimal), 2 (mild), 3 (moderate), 4 (severe). Two of the 12 items refer to dental care. The patient must be calm and sitting in a firm chair that doesn't have arms, and the patient cannot have anything in his or her mouth. The clinician asks the patient about the condition of his or her teeth and dentures, or if he or she is having any pain or discomfort from dentures.

The remaining 10 items refer to body movements themselves. In this section of the test, the clinician or rater asks the patient about body movements. The rater also looks at the patient in order to note any unusual movements first-hand. The patient is asked if he or she has noticed any unusual movements of the mouth, face, hands or feet. If the patient says yes, the clinician then asks if the movements annoy the patient or interfere with daily activities. Next, the patient is observed for any movements while sitting in the chair with feet flat on the floor, knees separated slightly with the hands on the knees. The patient is asked to open his or her mouth and stick out the tongue twice while the rater watches. The patient is then asked to tap his or her thumb with each finger very rapidly for 10–15 seconds, the right hand first and then the left hand. Again the rater observes the patient's face and legs for any abnormal movements.

After the face and hands have been tested, the patient is then asked to flex (bend) and extend one arm at a time. The patient is then asked to stand up so that the rater can observe the entire body for movements. Next, the patient is asked to extend both arms in front of the body with the palms facing downward. The trunk, legs and mouth are again observed for signs of TD. The patient then walks a few paces, while his or her gait and hands are observed by the rater twice.

RESULTS

The total score on the AIMS test is not reported to the patient. A rating of 2 or higher on the AIMS scale, however, is evidence of tardive dyskinesia. If the patient has mild TD in two areas or moderate movements in one area, then he or she should be given a diagnosis of TD. The AIMS test is considered extremely reliable when it is given by experienced raters.

If the patient's score on the AIMS test suggests the diagnosis of TD, the clinician must consider whether the patient still needs to be on an antipsychotic medication. This question should be discussed with the patient and his or her family. If the patient requires ongoing treatment with antipsychotic drugs, the dose can often be lowered. A lower dosage should result in a lower level of TD symptoms. Another option is to place the patient on a trial dosage of Clozapine (Clozaril), a newer antipsychotic medication that has fewer side effects than the older neuroleptics.

EXAMINATION PROCEDURE

Either before or after completing the examination procedure, observe the patient unobtrusively at rest (e.g., in the waiting room).

The chair to be used in this examination should be a hard, firm one without arms. Have the person remove their shoes and socks.

1. Ask the patient whether there is anything in his or her mouth (such as gum or candy) and, if so, to remove it.
2. Ask about the *current* condition of the patient's teeth. Ask if he or she wears dentures. Ask whether teeth or dentures bother the patient *now*.
3. Ask whether the patient notices any movements in his or her mouth, face, hands, or feet. If yes, ask the patient to describe them and to indicate to what extent they *currently* bother the patient or interfere with activities.
4. Have the patient sit in chair with hands on knees, legs slightly apart, and feet flat on floor. (Look at the entire body for movements while the patient is in this position.)
5. Ask the patient to sit with hands hanging unsupported—if male, between his legs, if female and wearing a dress, hanging over her knees. (Observe hands and other body areas).
6. Ask the patient to open his or her mouth. (Observe the tongue at rest within the mouth.) Do this twice.
7. Ask the patient to protrude his or her tongue. (Observe abnormalities of tongue movement.) Do this twice.

8. Ask the patient to tap his or her thumb with each finger as rapidly as possible for 10 to 15 seconds, first with right hand, then with left hand. (Observe facial and leg movements.)

9. Flex and extend the patient's left and right arms, one at a time.

10. Ask the patient to stand up. (Observe the patient in profile. Observe all body areas again, hips included.)

11. Ask the patient to extend both arms out in front, palms down. (Observe trunk, legs, and mouth.)

12. Have the patient walk a few paces, turn, and walk back to the chair. (Observe hands and gait.) Do this twice.

Abnormal Involuntary Movement Scale (117-AIMS). In: Guy W, ed. *ECDEU Assessment Manual for Psychopharmacology*. Rockville, MD: National Institute of Mental Health; 1976:534–537.

APPENDIX D: GUIDELINES FOR INFORMED CONSENT

We recommend that you include the following elements in your informed consent process:

- Diagnoses or working diagnoses.
- Target symptoms, prioritized.
- Proposed medication plan, including name of medication, dosage, timing, and plans for adjusting.
- Specific rationale (benefits) and risks (side effects).
- Alternatives to medication, including no medication.
- FDA-approved use vs off-label use of medication. This is central to much of pediatric psychopharmacology since so many of our medications are prescribed off-label. Families need to know that while doctors are allowed to use medications however they see fit, many medications are not approved by the FDA for children and are officially considered experimental. The discussion should include some information on common off-label uses, a sense of the supporting research and rationale, and a plan to manage problems if they arise.
- Any additional regulations, if applicable (eg, state or institutional requirements regarding use or follow-up).
- Cost of care, including medications, generics, follow-up visits, and cost-saving strategies.
- Monitoring plan, including labs and frequency of follow-up visits.
- Concurrent treatment and intervention: therapies, school plans, etc.
- Check your state laws for age of consent for mental health care, and specifically for medication treatment.
- For children whose parents are divorced, check the custody papers for information on shared health care decision making. For example, can one parent consent to medication if the other parent objects? There may also be a difference between routine and emergency situations.
- Consider assent: What will you tell the child, and to what extent can the child be a partner in the process?
- Agree to stay in contact as needed, and specify how to reach you or your coverage.
- Informed consent is an ongoing process that supports good care. Periodically document that the treatment plan was reviewed and that changes to the plan were made, if applicable.

APPENDIX E: DRUG INTERACTIONS IN PSYCHIATRY

Drug interactions can be one of the most challenging aspects of psychopharmacology. Today's psychiatrists often use complex medication regimens, while patients frequently take medications for multiple medical comorbidities. It's impossible to keep track of all of these, but it is important (1) to understand basic concepts of drug-drug interactions, (2) to know where to find information regarding such interactions, and (3) to know which interactions may be clinically relevant. This review is pertinent to both general and child psychiatry; however, see the General Tips chapter for specific thoughts on age-related differences in drug metabolism in children.

The majority of interactions in psychiatry will not result in a serious outcome. Many interactions, however, may result in decreased efficacy or increased adverse effects, and these can be easily avoided. And we often do not have data on side effects and interactions in children.

First, let's review some basic concepts. A drug interaction occurs when the pharmacologic action of one drug is altered by the co-administration of another drug. The two major types of drug interactions are **pharmacodynamic** (what the drug does to the body) and **pharmacokinetic** (what the body does to the drug). Pharmacodynamic interactions impact the effects of the drug at the target site. Pharmacokinetic interactions, on the other hand, impact the amount of time the drug stays in the body and its distribution to active sites.

Pharmacodynamic interactions take place at the level of neurotransmitters and receptors. For example, clonazepam (Klonopin) makes people sleepy by stimulating GABA receptors. Quetiapine (Seroquel) also makes people sleepy, probably by blocking histamine receptors. Combine the two, and patients become *really* sleepy. Pharmacodynamic interactions may also cause two drugs to *oppose* one another. Many of the dementia medications, for example, increase acetylcholine levels, while many psychiatric medications have primary (eg, benztropine) or secondary (eg, clozapine) anticholinergic effects. Giving both together may negate the beneficial effects of the dementia medication.

Some notable—and potentially dangerous—pharmacodynamic interactions in psychiatry include serotonin syndrome (too many serotonergic agents used together); the MAOI-type hypertensive crisis (MAOIs taken with foods high in tyramine); and arrhythmia-causing combinations (medications that increase QT interval, when taken together, may cause life-threatening arrhythmias, such as torsades de pointes). We often try to avoid these problems by doing things like lowering doses or choosing alternative medications. In such cases, we're trying to avoid pharmacodynamic interactions.

Pharmacokinetic interactions are harder to predict, since they are often non-intuitive and are unrelated to the pharmacologic action of drugs. Pharmacokinetic interactions depend on where and when two or more drugs come in contact during drug processing. Drugs can interact with one another at four different junctures:

- Absorption (getting the drug into the bloodstream)
- Distribution (ferrying drugs to different tissues once they've been absorbed)
- Excretion (sending drugs into the sewage system)
- Metabolism (dismantling drugs into simpler components)

We'll discuss each one in turn, focusing on some common examples in psychopharmacology.

Absorption. Drug-food, rather than drug-drug, interactions are most relevant during absorption. For example, ziprasidone (Geodon) and lurasidone (Latuda) absorption are both decreased by 50%–60% when taken without food, which is why we instruct our patients to take these drugs after a full meal (at least, we *should* be doing this!). Food also speeds absorption of both sertraline (Zoloft) and quetiapine, but only by 25% or so, usually not enough to be clinically relevant. Meanwhile, food famously *slows* absorption of erectile dysfunction drugs such as sildenafil (Viagra) and vardenafil (Levitra)—but not tadalafil (Cialis).

Distribution. Valproic acid (Depakote) is highly protein-bound, and only the unbound portion (the "free fraction") of the drug has a therapeutic effect. Aspirin is also highly protein-bound, so if your patient combines the two drugs, the aspirin will kick some of the valproic acid off its protein—mainly albumin—which would cause the free fraction of the drug to increase. Standard valproic acid levels in the lab usually do not distinguish between free and bound fractions, so a serum level might be normal, even though the actual functioning valproic acid can be very high—and this could cause side effects. One way to check for this interaction is to order a free valproate level; the normal therapeutic range is about 5 mcg/mL–10 mcg/mL, much less than the total valproic acid therapeutic range of about 40 mcg/mL–100 mcg/mL.

Excretion. Lithium, unlike almost all other drugs in psychiatry, is not metabolized. Instead, it is excreted unchanged in the urine. Because of this, liver disease does not affect lithium levels, but changes in kidney function will affect such levels. Caffeine, for example, speeds up kidney function and can reduce lithium levels. On the other hand, ibuprofen (along with other NSAIDs) and ACE inhibitors decrease lithium excretion, increase lithium levels, and could potentially cause toxic effects. Other psychiatric medications that are not metabolized by the liver and rather excreted by the kidneys are gabapentin (Neurontin), pregabalin (Lyrica), and paliperidone (Invega).

Liver metabolism. Most drug-drug interactions take place in the liver, where drugs are processed in order to render them water-soluble so that the body can excrete them via the urine or feces. There are two phases of liver metabolism. Phase

I involves the famous cytochrome P-450 enzymes, or CYP450. These enzymes attack drugs in a variety of ways, such as hydroxylation (adding a hydroxyl group), dealkylation (taking away an alkyl group), and several others. Unfortunately for those of us trying to remember drug interactions, there are many subfamilies of CYP450 enzymes: CYP1A2, 2B6, 2C9, 2C19, 2D6, 3A4, and several others. Phase II metabolism continues the process of biotransformation, relying mainly on glucuronidation—which is rarely a factor in drug interactions in psychiatric practice.

Practical Implications of Drug-Drug Interactions

To understand drug-drug interactions, you'll need to refamiliarize yourself with some basic terms. Drugs are **substrates** of specific enzymes (the medication relies on that/those enzymatic pathway(s) for metabolism). An **inhibitor** is a drug that binds more tightly to an enzyme than the usual substrate and prevents the enzyme from doing its job; as a result, the substrate for that enzyme gets stuck in a game of musical chairs as it scurries around looking for a free enzyme system to break it down. Since this drug is not getting metabolized as quickly as it otherwise would (the inhibitor is preventing it from doing so), its serum levels become higher than expected. On the other hand, **inducers** stimulate the production of extra enzymes. With more enzymes around, the substrate for that enzyme is broken down more rapidly, leading to lower serum drug levels.

Now that you know the basics, how can you most efficiently apply them to your practice? Here are some suggestions.

- Identify the 10 drugs that you most commonly prescribe, and memorize the major drug interactions for each one.
- Antidepressants, antipsychotics, antibiotics, antiretrovirals, and older anticonvulsants have a high likelihood of significant drug interactions—so be particularly vigilant if your patient is taking any of these.
- Recognize the drugs with a narrow therapeutic window (ie, when the toxic dose is not much higher than the therapeutic dose). Commonly used drugs with narrow therapeutic windows include lithium, carbamazepine (Tegretol), warfarin (Coumadin), digoxin (Lanoxin), phenytoin (Dilantin), and phenobarbital.
- Recognize drugs that cause serious side effects and outcomes if blood levels are significantly increased or decreased (eg, oral contraceptives, lamotrigine, clozapine, TCAs, warfarin).
- Drugs with long half-lives, such as diazepam (Valium) or aripiprazole (Abilify), can be particularly troublesome when involved in drug interactions, because metabolic inhibitors—or hepatic dysfunction—can make them ultra-long-lasting. Be cautious with any new or rarely prescribed drugs: Neither you nor anybody else has had much experience with them, and unreported drug interactions can appear.
- The risk of drug interactions can increase exponentially as the number of drugs increases. Setting a threshold to check for interactions is helpful (eg, any patient on 3 or more drugs).

Another important concern with drug interactions is timing. *Inhibition* happens quickly. It can occur with the first dose of a medication and can subside quickly. How long it takes to subside depends on the inhibitor's half-life. Generally, the inhibition will stop after 5 half-lives of the inhibitor drug. On the other hand, for *induction* to occur, the body has to synthesize more CYP450 enzymes, and this can take up to 4 weeks. This accounts for the delayed "auto-induction" of carbamazepine. Likewise, for induction to subside, these extra enzymes need to be broken down, a process that could also take several weeks. As a general rule, any drug prescribed with its inhibitor should be started at half the usual dose and titrated more slowly. Conversely, a drug prescribed with its inducer may need to be dosed higher after the few weeks it takes for induction to occur.

Useful References for Drug Interactions

It's ideal to have a useful resource to look up interaction information. Keeping track of interactions has become less daunting with the advent of free software from companies like Epocrates (www.epocrates.com) and Medscape (www.medscape.com), which allow you to check for potential interactions among all possible combinations of drugs.

But there are various problems with the computerized databases you'll find at these sites or in your electronic prescribing system (if you have one). For one, the databases tend to be overly inclusive, often listing every conceivable interaction, no matter how unlikely. As an example, citalopram (Celexa), an SSRI considered by most of us to be a pretty safe choice in combination with just about any drug, looks pretty dangerous in the Epocrates database. Moreover, these databases are often populated with drug-class information rather than medication-specific information, making important nuances unavailable to the user. That's where your clinical judgment and experience come in!

Free
- Medscape (www.medscape.com/druginfo/druginterchecker)
- http://www.epocrates.com (you'll need to register first)
- https://www.drugs.com/drug_interactions.html
- http://medicine.iupui.edu/clinpharm/ddis
- https://www.rxlist.com

Not free

- Lexi-Interact (http://bit.ly/fugKmk), $75 for a 1-year subscription

We also provide a table, "CYP450 Drug Interactions for Some Commonly Prescribed Medications," on the following pages for your reference (adapted from Goren J & Carlat D, *The Carlat Psychiatry Report* 2011;9(2):1–5).

Appendix E continued on the next page.

APPENDIX E: Drug Interactions in Psychiatry

CYP450 Family	Inducers	Inhibitors	Substrates ("Victim" Drugs)	Symptoms When Induced	Symptoms When Inhibited
1A2	Armodafinil Carbamazepine Cigarette smoke Modafinil Omeprazole Rifampin Ritonavir St. John's wort	Ciprofloxacin Fluvoxamine Melatonin Norfloxacin	Asenapine	Loss of efficacy (psychosis)	Insomnia/EPS
			Caffeine	Withdrawal headaches	Jitteriness
			Clozapine	Loss of efficacy (psychosis)	Seizures/sedation/anticholinergic effects
			Duloxetine	Loss of efficacy (depression)	Increased blood pressure
			Fluvoxamine	Loss of efficacy (depression/OCD)	GI/sedation
			Melatonin	Loss of efficacy (insomnia)	Sedation
			Mirtazapine	Loss of efficacy (depression)	Sedation
			Olanzapine	Loss of efficacy (psychosis)	Sedation
			Ramelteon	Loss of efficacy (insomnia)	Sedation
			Tasimelteon	Loss of efficacy (insomnia)	Sedation
			Thiothixene	Loss of efficacy (psychosis)	EPS
			Trifluoperazine	Loss of efficacy (psychosis)	EPS
2B6	Carbamazepine Phenobarbital Phenytoin Rifampin	Clopidogrel Ketoconazole Ticlopidine	Bupropion	Loss of efficacy (depression)	Seizures/jitteriness/insomnia
			Methadone	Opiate withdrawal	CNS and respiratory depression
			Selegiline	Loss of efficacy (depression)	Insomnia/diarrhea
2C9	Barbiturates Carbamazepine Rifampin St. John's wort	Fluconazole Fluoxetine Fluvoxamine Isoniazid Metronidazole	Methadone	Opiate withdrawal	CNS and respiratory depression
			NSAIDs	Loss of pain control	GI effects
			Oral hypoglycemics	Loss of glycemic control	Hypoglycemia
			Warfarin	Loss of anticoagulant efficacy	Increased bleeding
2C19	Barbiturates Carbamazepine Rifampin	Fluconazole Fluoxetine Fluvoxamine Modafinil Oxcarbazepine	Barbiturates	Loss of efficacy (insomnia/anxiety/seizures)	Sedation/barbiturate intoxication
			Citalopram	Loss of efficacy (depression/anxiety)	GI effects
			Diazepam	Loss of efficacy (insomnia/anxiety/seizures)	Sedation/BZD intoxication
			Doxepin	Loss of efficacy (depression/anxiety/ insomnia)	Seizures/arrhythmia/anticholinergic effects
			Escitalopram	Loss of efficacy (depression/anxiety)	GI effects
			Methadone	Opiate withdrawal	CNS and respiratory depression
			Sertraline	Loss of efficacy (depression/anxiety)	GI effects

( ) indicates less potent inhibitory effect, therefore generally less of a risk except at higher dose

CYP450 Family	Inducers	Inhibitors	Substrates ("Victim" Drugs)	Symptoms When Induced	Symptoms When Inhibited
2D6	Not inducible	Asenapine Bupropion Duloxetine Fluoxetine Haloperidol Methadone Paroxetine (Perphenazine) Thioridazine Venlafaxine	Amphetamine	N/A	Insomnia/decreased appetite
			Aripiprazole	N/A	Akathisia/sedation
			Atomoxetine	N/A	GI/constipation
			Brexpiprazole	N/A	Akathisia/sedation
			Chlorpromazine	N/A	Seizures/sedation/anticholinergic effects
			Clozapine	N/A	Seizures/sedation/anticholinergic effects
			Codeine/hydrocodone	N/A	Less/no analgesia (not converted to morphine)
			Dextroamphetamine	N/A	Insomnia/decreased appetite
			Diphenhydramine	N/A	Sedation/anticholinergic effects
			Donepezil	N/A	GI effects
			Doxepin	N/A	Sedation/anticholinergic effects
			Doxylamine	N/A	Sedation/anticholinergic effects
			Duloxetine	N/A	Increased BP
			Fluoxetine	N/A	GI effects
			Fluphenazine	N/A	EPS
			Fluvoxamine	N/A	GI effects/sedation
			Galantamine	N/A	GI effects
			Haloperidol	N/A	EPS
			Iloperidone	N/A	Tachycardia/hypotension/stiffness
			Loxapine	N/A	EPS/sedation
			Methamphetamine	N/A	Insomnia/decreased appetite
			Mirtazapine	N/A	Somnolence
			Mixed amphetamine salts	N/A	Insomnia/decreased appetite
			Paroxetine	N/A	GI effects/anticholinergic effects/sedation
			Perphenazine	N/A	EPS/sedation
			Propranolol	N/A	Decreased BP/pulse
			Risperidone	N/A	EPS/orthostasis
			Thioridazine	N/A	Seizures/sedation/anticholinergic effects/QT prolongation
			Trazodone	N/A	Sedation
			Tricyclics	N/A	Seizures/arrhythmia/anticholinergic effects
			Venlafaxine	N/A	GI effects
			Vortioxetine	N/A	GI effects

( ) indicates less potent inhibitory effect, therefore generally less of a risk except at higher dose

CYP450 Family	Inducers	Inhibitors	Substrates ("Victim" Drugs)	Symptoms When Induced	Symptoms When Inhibited
3A4	Armodafinil Barbiturates Carbamazepine Modafinil Oxcarbazepine Phenytoin Rifampin St. John's wort (Topiramate)	Clarithromycin Fluconazole Fluvoxamine Grapefruit juice Ketoconazole Protease inhibitors	Alprazolam	Loss of efficacy (insomnia/anxiety/seizures)	Sedation/BZD intoxication
			Aripiprazole	Loss of efficacy (psychosis)	Akathisia/sedation
			Armodafinil	Loss of efficacy (narcolepsy)	Insomnia/increased pulse
			Avanafil	Loss of efficacy (sexual dysfunction)	Headache/flushing/prolonged erection
			Brexpiprazole	Loss of efficacy (psychosis)	Akathisia/sedation
			Buprenorphine	Opiate withdrawal	CNS and respiratory depression
			Buspirone	Loss of efficacy (anxiety)	GI effects/jitteriness
			Calcium channel blockers	Loss of efficacy (hypertension)	Hypotension
			Carbamazepine	Loss of efficacy/seizures	Sedation/arrhythmia
			Cariprazine	Loss of efficacy (psychosis)	Akathisia/sedation
			Citalopram	Loss of efficacy (depression/anxiety)	GI effects
			Clonazepam	Loss of efficacy (insomnia/anxiety/seizures)	Sedation/BZD intoxication
			Clozapine	Loss of efficacy (psychosis)	Seizures/sedation/anticholinergic effects
			Diazepam	Loss of efficacy (insomnia/anxiety/seizures)	Sedation/BZD intoxication
			Donepezil	Loss of efficacy (dementia)	GI effects
			Escitalopram	Loss of efficacy (depression/anxiety)	GI effects
			Eszopiclone	Loss of efficacy (insomnia)	Sedation/confusion
			Flibanserin	Loss of efficacy (sexual desire)	Nausea/dizziness/sedation
			Flurazepam	Loss of efficacy (insomnia)	Sedation/BZD intoxication
			Galantamine	Loss of efficacy (dementia)	GI effects
			Guanfacine	Loss of efficacy (ADHD)	Sedation/dry mouth/dizziness
			Iloperidone	Loss of efficacy (psychosis)	Sedation/dizziness
			Levomilnacipran	Loss of efficacy (depression)	GI effects
			Loxapine	Loss of efficacy (psychosis)	EPS/sedation
			Lurasidone	Loss of efficacy (psychosis)	Sedation/akathisia
			Methadone	Opiate withdrawal	CNS and respiratory depression
			Mirtazapine	Loss of efficacy (depression/insomnia)	Somnolence
			Modafinil	Loss of efficacy (narcolepsy)	Insomnia/increased pulse
			Oral contraceptives	Loss of efficacy (pregnancy)	GI effects
			Pimavanserin	Loss of efficacy (psychosis)	Nausea/confusion
			Quetiapine	Loss of efficacy (psychosis)	Sedation/orthostasis
			Statins (not pravastatin)	Loss of efficacy (hyperlipidemia)	Rhabdomyolysis

( ) indicates less potent inhibitory effect, therefore generally less of a risk except at higher dose

CYP450 Family	Inducers	Inhibitors	Substrates ("Victim" Drugs)	Symptoms When Induced	Symptoms When Inhibited
3A4	Armodafinil Barbiturates Carbamazepine Modafinil Oxcarbazepine Phenytoin Rifampin St. John's wort (Topiramate)	Clarithromycin Fluconazole Fluvoxamine Grapefruit juice Ketoconazole Protease inhibitors	Sildenafil	Loss of efficacy (sexual dysfunction)	Headache/flushing/prolonged erection
			Suvorexant	Loss of efficacy (insomnia)	Sedation/confusion
			Tadalafil	Loss of efficacy (sexual dysfunction)	Headache/flushing/prolonged erection
			Tasimelteon	Loss of efficacy (insomnia)	Sedation
			Tiagabine	Loss of efficacy (seizures)	Dizziness/somnolence/difficulty concentrating
			Trazodone	Loss of efficacy (insomnia)	Sedation/orthostasis
			Triazolam	Loss of efficacy (insomnia/anxiety/seizures)	Sedation/BZD intoxication
			Tricyclics	Loss of efficacy (depression/anxiety)	Seizures/arrhythmia/anticholinergic effects
			Vardenafil	Loss of efficacy (sexual dysfunction)	Headache/flushing/prolonged erection
			Vilazodone	Loss of efficacy (depression/anxiety)	GI effects
			Zaleplon	Loss of efficacy (insomnia)	Sedation/confusion
			Ziprasidone	Loss of efficacy (psychosis)	Sedation/akathisia
			Zolpidem	Loss of efficacy (insomnia)	Sedation/confusion

( ) indicates less potent inhibitory effect, therefore generally less of a risk except at higher dose

APPENDIX F: SCHEDULES OF CONTROLLED SUBSTANCES

In 1970, under the Controlled Substance Act, the FDA created classification schedules that organize drugs into groups based on their risk of abuse or harm. There are 5 classifications of controlled substances (Schedule I, II, III, IV, and V), and drugs with the highest risk-to-benefit ratio are considered Schedule I drugs. Most drugs used in psychiatry are not scheduled at all (antidepressants, antipsychotics, etc). Some of us get confused about whether the most restricted drugs are Schedule I or V. Here's a mnemonic: The number 1 looks like a needle, and a needle is used to inject heroin—which is the prototypical Schedule I drug.

Prescription drug monitoring programs (PDMPs) are searchable databases that can help prescribers identify potential abuse or diversion of controlled substances. If you prescribe controlled substances like benzodiazepines and stimulants, it's a good idea to learn about your state's PDMP laws, consider your search results in the context of all available information, and watch for regulatory changes over the next few years. For example, since October 2, 2018, prescribers in California are required to check the state CURES database before prescribing controlled substances. To find your state's program, check with the PDMP Training and Technical Assistance Center (http://www.pdmpassist.org/content/state-pdmp-websites).

Schedule	Description	Prescribing Implications	Some Examples
I	No accepted medical use, high potential for abuse, illegal to possess or use	Can't be prescribed at all (with the exception of medical marijuana in some states)	Heroin, LSD, ecstasy, and others Marijuana (though legalized in some states, it is still illegal at the federal level)
II	High potential for abuse, but legal for medical use	Can be prescribed only 1 month at a time, cannot be refilled, cannot be called in, and patient must give pharmacy a paper script (unless you use an e-prescribing program that is certified by DEA to allow prescribing of controlled substances)	All psychostimulants, such as amphetamine and methylphenidate Opiates that are especially potent, such as oxycodone, fentanyl, and others Vicodin (hydrocodone and acetaminophen)—recently reclassified from Schedule III to Schedule II
III	Lower potential for abuse than Schedule I or II, but still pretty abusable	Can be refilled up to 5 times (no more than 6 months), can be called in	Suboxone (buprenorphine/naloxone) Ketamine Xyrem (sodium oxybate) Anabolic steroids Barbiturates Dronabinol (Marinol)
IV	Lower potential for abuse than Schedule III	Can be refilled up to 5 times (no more than 6 months), can be called in	All benzodiazepines (eg, clonazepam, lorazepam, etc) Various hypnotics, such as zolpidem, zaleplon, and suvorexant (Belsomra) Wake-promoting agents, like modafinil and armodafinil Tramadol (Ultram) Carisoprodol (Soma) Lorcaserin (Belviq), an anti-obesity drug
V	Lowest potential for abuse	Can be refilled as many times as prescriber chooses (eg, for 1 year or more), can be called in	Pregabalin (Lyrica) Cough preparations with small amounts of codeine, such as Robitussin AC Antidiarrheal Lomotil (diphenoxylate/atropine)

An updated and more complete list of the schedules is published annually in Title 21 *Code of Federal Regulations* and can be found here: www.deadiversion.usdoj.gov/21cfr/cfr/2108cfrt.htm

APPENDIX G: LAB MONITORING FOR PSYCHIATRIC MEDICATIONS

This is a short and sweet table listing the medications that most psychiatrists would agree require lab monitoring. Our recommendations are quite abbreviated, and we haven't spelled out whether you should order labs before or after starting the medications, nor how you should do follow-up monitoring. There's just too much variation in practice for us to give authoritative detailed guidelines. These medications are mainly here to jog your memory, so you don't forget to at least consider what type of monitoring to do.

Medications	Recommended Laboratory Tests
Acamprosate	BUN/creatinine if renal impairment is suspected
Amantadine	BUN/creatinine if renal impairment is suspected
Antipsychotics—second generation, primarily clozapine, aripiprazole, olanzapine, quetiapine, paliperidone, risperidone[1]	BMI, fasting glucose and lipids; for quetiapine consider periodic slit-lamp examinations
Atomoxetine	LFTs
Carbamazepine	CBZ level, complete blood count (CBC), sodium, LFTs, pregnancy test, HLA-B*1502 in Asians[2]
Chlorpromazine	BMI, ECG if cardiac disease, fasting glucose and lipids
Citalopram	ECG if cardiac disease, dose ≥40 mg/day
Clozapine	BMI, fasting glucose and lipids, CBC (REMS system required in US)
Desvenlafaxine	Periodic BP
Deutetrabenazine	ECG if cardiac disease
Disulfiram	LFTs if liver disease is suspected
Duloxetine	LFTs if liver disease is suspected[3]
Gabapentin	BUN/creatinine if renal impairment is suspected
Levomilnacipran	Periodic BP/pulse rate
Lithium	BMI, Li level, TSH, BUN/creatinine[4], pregnancy test, ECG if cardiac disease
Methadone	ECG if cardiac disease
Mirtazapine	BMI, fasting glucose and lipids
Naltrexone	LFTs if liver disease is suspected
Oxcarbazepine	Sodium, HLA-B*1502 in Asians[5]
Paliperidone	BMI, prolactin if symptoms, fasting glucose and lipids
Pregabalin	BUN/creatinine if renal impairment is suspected
Risperidone	BMI, prolactin if symptoms, fasting glucose and lipids
SSRIs	Sodium in elderly if fatigue, dizziness, confusion
Stimulants	Periodic BP/P, height and weight, ECG if cardiac disease
Thioridazine	BMI, ECG if cardiac disease, fasting glucose and lipids
Topiramate	Bicarbonate
Tricyclic antidepressants	ECG if cardiac disease
Valbenazine	ECG if cardiac disease
Valproic acid	BMI, VPA level, LFTs, CBC for platelets, pregnancy test, ammonia if confusion
Venlafaxine	Periodic BP
Ziprasidone	BMI, ECG if cardiac disease, fasting glucose and lipids

[1] Some guidelines recommend monitoring glucose and lipids with all SGAs.

[2] HLA-B*1502 is a gene that increases the risk of developing toxic epidermal necrolysis (TEN) and Stevens-Johnson syndrome (SJS) in response to taking carbamazepine. Asians, especially the Han Chinese, are much more likely to have the gene than other populations.

[3] Duloxetine should not be prescribed in patients with significant alcohol use or evidence of chronic liver disease as it can lead to hepatic failure in rare cases (Cymbalta prescribing information). While the manufacturer does not recommend baseline LFTs for all patients, some clinicians do so anyway to be extra cautious.

[4] The serum creatinine is used to compute the estimated glomerular filtration rate (eGFR), a more precise measure of kidney functioning. Increasingly, laboratory test results include the estimated GFR. You can calculate it yourself using an online calculator at https://www.niddk.nih.gov/health-information/communication-programs/nkdep/laboratory-evaluation/glomerular-filtration-rate-calculators.

[5] HLA-B*1502 is a gene that increases the risk of developing toxic epidermal necrolysis (TEN) and Stevens-Johnson syndrome (SJS) in response to taking carbamazepine. Asians, especially the Han Chinese, are much more likely to have the gene than other populations.

APPENDIX H: PHARMACOGENETIC TESTING RECOMMENDATIONS

THE BASICS

Variations in patients' genetic profiles can affect how they respond to medications. While the actual clinical importance of this phenomenon is not yet clear, it's likely that genetic variations in pharmacokinetic genes have some effect on serum levels of medications in many patients. Based on these CYP450 polymorphisms, individuals are categorized in different ways with respect to specific enzymes:

Extensive metabolizers: Otherwise known as "normal" metabolizers, these people have normally active CYP450 genes on both chromosomes, meaning that they see an average level of drug in the body.

Intermediate metabolizers: These people metabolize drugs a bit more slowly than extensive metabolizers, but not dramatically so.

Poor metabolizers: These people carry inactive or partially active CYP450 genes, and therefore metabolize drugs significantly more slowly than extensive metabolizers. This may result in more side effects since serum drug levels are higher.

Ultrarapid metabolizers: With extra copies of certain genes, these people metabolize drugs more quickly than extensive metabolizers, sometimes requiring unusually high doses of medications to achieve a therapeutic level.

There are also genetic variations in pharmacodynamic genes that might increase or decrease the efficacy of drugs, but the evidence for this effect is less robust than for pharmacokinetic effects.

PHARMACOGENETIC TESTING IN CLINICAL PRACTICE

The science of pharmacogenetic testing is complex, which makes it hard for us mere mortals to evaluate the claims of the many commercial test kits flooding the market.

In March 2017, *The Carlat Psychiatry Report* explored this topic and focused on three tests: Genesight, Genecept, and CNSDose. We concluded that the evidence was not yet robust enough to recommend any of these tests. However, we did review information from FDA drug labels and created a table listing FDA recommendations for pharmacogenetic testing relevant to specific psychotropic drugs.

Many of the recommendations are to lower starting doses in patients who are poor metabolizers. For example, in aripiprazole's label, you'll read: "Dosing recommendation in patients who are classified as CYP450 2D6 poor metabolizers (PM): The aripiprazole dose in PM patients should initially be reduced to one-half (50%) of the usual dose and then adjusted to achieve a favorable clinical response."

While the FDA does not specifically ask you to order genetic testing, you will not know whether your patient is a poor metabolizer unless someone has ordered it. Therefore, a case could be made for selectively ordering CYP450 testing to ensure you dose drugs in accordance with FDA labeling. Whether you do this is a judgment call; most of us are content to skip the genetic testing, and instead choose to start most medications at a low dose and titrate up gradually in order to prevent side effects.

APPENDIX H: FDA Label Information Relevant to Pharmacogenetic Testing for Psychiatric Drugs

Medication	FDA Recommendations	Clinical Rationale
Aripiprazole Atomoxetine Brexpiprazole Iloperidone Perphenazine Vortioxetine	Reduce dose in CYP2D6 PMs.[1]	Usual starting dose is too high in PMs, so start lower and increase gradually.
Amitriptyline Clomipramine Clozapine Desipramine Doxepin Imipramine Nortriptyline Protriptyline Trimipramine	Monitor levels in CYP2D6 PMs.	These medications, most of which are tricyclic antidepressants, can cause life-threatening side effects if levels are too high. Consider monitoring serum levels in PMs.
Citalopram	Maximum recommended daily dose of 20 mg (rather than 40 mg) for CYP2C19 PMs.	Risk of QT prolongation and cardiac arrhythmia.
Thioridazine	Contraindicated in CYP2D6 PMs, due to risk of QT prolongation.	Risk of QT prolongation and cardiac arrhythmia.
Pimozide	In CYP2D6 PMs, dose should not exceed 4 mg/day in adults.	Risk of QT prolongation and cardiac arrhythmia.
Carbamazepine Oxcarbazepine	Avoid or use cautiously in individuals with the HLA-B*1502 allele (applicable to Asians).	Risk of serious rashes such as Stevens-Johnson syndrome.

[1] PM = poor metabolizer

Source: http://www.fda.gov/Drugs/ScienceResearch/ResearchAreas/Pharmacogenetics/ucm083378.htm

APPENDIX I: MEDICATIONS IN PREGNANCY AND LACTATION RISK INFORMATION

By way of explanation, we elected to include this appendix because some of our teen patients become pregnant, as do some of the mothers of our pediatric patients, during their mental health treatment. Many of us treat women of childbearing age in any case. Determining the risk of medications in pregnancy used to be a simple matter of looking up a drug's pregnancy categorization in the *PDR*. This ranged from category "A," which is the lowest risk, to "X," which means the drug is contraindicated in pregnancy. But this ABCDX system provided very little practical or clinically useful information. In 2014, the FDA came up with a new system of labeling, which requires descriptive subsections on different aspects of pregnancy and lactation, and omits the letter categories—though you'll still see the old system in use for drugs approved before 2015.

Pregnancy presents a unique problem to the psychiatrist. Contrary to what many may think or assume, pregnancy does not protect a woman from an acute episode, a recurrence, or an exacerbation of psychiatric illness. Withholding medications during pregnancy can *sometimes* be an appropriate option, but this is generally not recommended. Ever-mounting research demonstrates that the mental well-being of the mother during pregnancy and in the postpartum period (and beyond) is critical to the emotional development of the child. And since all psychotropic medications cross the placenta to at least *some* degree, their potential effects on the fetus, on labor and delivery, and on the neonate must be considered and balanced with the risk of *not* treating the mother with medication (see our July/August 2016 double issue of *The Carlat Psychiatry Report* for an overview). A similar risk-benefit assessment must be considered in the case of a mother who wishes to breastfeed her child, as psychotropic medications are excreted into breast milk to varying degrees.

One of us (TP) is a pharmacist specializing in psychopharmacology, and commonly consulted by psychiatrists to provide updated information on the safety of medications in pregnancy and breastfeeding. It is a difficult task, because the quantity and quality of data vary greatly. The accompanying table was developed by pulling together a variety of sources, including isolated case reports, case series, birth registries, retrospective surveys, prospective comparative cohort studies, case control studies, and meta-analyses. Making judgments about which medication to use—or not use—in a pregnant or lactating woman is a delicate balancing act, involving an assessment of the severity of the underlying illness vs the uncertainties inherent in prescribing medications when the available data are limited.

In reading the table, keep the following in mind: In the general US population, the baseline rate of major malformations is between 1% and 4%, depending on the population studied and the definitions of "malformations" used. If treatment is necessary, monotherapy with the lowest *effective* dose and for the shortest duration is prudent. Safety data are generally more robust with older agents, and for that reason older agents—with a few key exceptions—are more preferable than newer drugs with less established safety profiles.

Almost all drugs enter breast milk. The exposure to the infant is described as a percentage of the maternal dose—that is, how much of the weight-adjusted maternal dose is actually excreted into the breast milk. When less than 10% of a mother's dose of medication is excreted into the breast milk, it is generally considered compatible with breastfeeding (with some exceptions) since these low serum levels are unlikely to lead to adverse effects in the infant.

While the table summarizes the current knowledge about psychotropic medication in pregnancy and lactation, information in this area is constantly evolving. If you regularly treat women of childbearing age, we suggest that you keep up with new data, consult with experts, and use resources such as the Organization of Teratology Information Specialists at www.mothertobaby.org or 866-626-6847; Motherisk at www.motherisk.org; or the LactMed peer-reviewed database of the National Library of Medicine, updated monthly at http://1.usa.gov/15eWNH. Another good resource is the MGH Center for Women's Mental Health at www.womensmentalhealth.org. And, if you don't mind paying a fee (or if you are a trainee and have free access), you can check out www.reprotox.org, an online database of summaries. Another source of information can be the drug labeling, which, as of 2015, is more detailed than in the past. These resources, along with our table, provide information based upon the available evidence (or lack thereof), but the ultimate clinical decision comes down to careful and individualized consideration between the physician and the patient and her family.

Additional References

- Besag FM. ADHD treatment and pregnancy. *Drug Saf* 2014;37(6):397–408.
- Chisolm MS et al. Management of psychotropic drugs during pregnancy. *BMJ* 2016;352:h5918.
- Khan SJ et al. Bipolar disorder in pregnancy and postpartum: Principles of management. *Curr Psychiatry Rep* 2016;18(2):13.
- McLafferty LP et al. Guidelines for the management of pregnant women with substance use disorders. *Psychosomatics* 2016;57(2):115–130.
- Muzik M et al. Use of antidepressants during pregnancy? What to consider when weighing treatment with antidepressants against untreated depression. *Matern Child Health J* 2016;20(11):2268–2279.
- Ornoy A et al. Antidepressant, antipsychotics, and mood stabilizers in pregnancy: What do we know and how should we treat pregnant women with depression? *Birth Defects Res* 2017;109(12):933–956.
- Oyebode F et al. Psychotropics in pregnancy: Safety and other considerations. *Pharmacol Ther* 2012;135(1):71–77.

- Payne JL. Psychopharmacology in pregnancy and breastfeeding. *Psychiatr Clin North Am* 2017;40(2):217–238.
- Rowe H et al. Maternal medication, drug use, and breastfeeding. *Child Adolesc Psychiatr Clin N Am* 2015;24(1):1–20.
- Sachs HC et al. The transfer of drugs and therapeutics into human breast milk: An update on selected topics. *Pediatrics* 2013;132(3):e796–e809.
- Vigod S et al. Depression in pregnancy. *BMJ* 2016;352:i547.

Appendix I continued on the next page.

APPENDIX I: Medications in Pregnancy and Lactation Risk Information

Medication	Pregnancy	Breastfeeding	Recommendations
Anxiolytics/hypnotics			
Benzodiazepines (various agents)	Possible increased incidence of cleft lip or palate (with first trimester exposure); floppy infant syndrome (with exposure just before delivery); neonatal withdrawal syndrome; lower Apgar scores	Excretion varies with different benzodiazepines, but it is always less than 10%. Excessive sedation in infant, lethargy with consequent feeding difficulty and weight loss reported.	Try to avoid use in first trimester and late in pregnancy (although intermittent use less likely to induce withdrawal symptoms in neonate). Lorazepam (Ativan) may be best in class to use due to lack of active metabolites and relatively shorter half-life. Monitor sedation in breastfed infants; use of shorter-acting agents preferred.
Buspirone (BuSpar)	Fewer data; difficult to determine risks	Low to undetectable infant levels reported	Due to lack of data, other agents with larger safety database should be considered first
Diphenhydramine (Benadryl)	Fairly consistent data show lack of associated malformations	Larger doses or more prolonged use may cause adverse effects in the infant	Considered to be the safest hypnotic in pregnancy and breastfeeding
Non-benzodiazepines: Eszopiclone (Lunesta) Zaleplon (Sonata) Zolpidem (Ambien)	Fewer data show no increased risk of malformations	Relatively low levels in breast milk. Most data are with zolpidem. Zolpidem is relatively hydrophilic and excreted rapidly; therefore, may be favored.	Reserve for second-line use due to paucity of data. If unavoidable, use zolpidem at lowest dose possible.
Suvorexant (Belsomra)	No data	No data	Best to use other agents with data and longer record of experience
Trazodone	Fewer data show no increased risk of malformations	<1% excretion; not expected to cause adverse effects in breastfed infants	Probably safe
Mood stabilizers			
Carbamazepine (Tegretol)	Rate of major malformation reported to be 2.2%–7.9%. Neural tube defects (0.5%–1%), craniofacial defects, cardiovascular malformations, and hypospadias reported.	Relatively high levels in breast milk but with few adverse effects reported. Sedation, poor sucking, withdrawal reactions, and 3 cases of hepatic dysfunction have been reported.	Avoid if possible. High-dose (4 mg) folic acid supplementation recommended.
Lamotrigine (Lamictal)	Rate of major malformations reported to be 1%–5.6%. Increased risk of oral clefts (0.4%).	Based on limited data, thought to be safe; however, infant exposure can be high and can vary widely (reports of 18%–60% of maternal concentrations); monitor infant. Relatively high infant exposure (22.7%); avoid or exercise caution.	Considered to be the safest of the anticonvulsants in pregnancy, though good safety data are sparse
Lithium (Eskalith, Lithobid)	Rate of major malformations reported to be 4%–12%. Increased risk of cardiovascular malformation, Ebstein's anomaly; risk is lower than previously thought (0.05%–0.1%). Increased maternal risk of diabetes, polyhydramnios, thyroid dysfunction during pregnancy.	30%–50% excretion; not recommended due to high risk of toxicity	Avoid, particularly in first trimester. Check serum levels and thyroid function frequently during pregnancy. Changes in metabolism and total body water necessitate frequent dose adjustment, particularly in third trimester. Avoid in breastfeeding if possible.
Oxcarbazepine (Trileptal)	Unlike carbamazepine, there is no epoxide metabolite formed, so oxcarbazepine may be less teratogenic; a Danish study showed no increased risk of major malformation. However, data with oxcarbazepine are limited.	Limited information suggests oxcarbazepine would not be expected to cause adverse effects in breastfed infants, especially if the infant is older than 2 months. Monitor infant for drowsiness, adequate weight gain, and developmental milestones, especially in younger, exclusively breastfed infants and when using combinations of anticonvulsants.	Use caution until more data available

Medication	Pregnancy	Breastfeeding	Recommendations
Valproate (Depakote)	Most teratogenic of all mood stabilizers, with a 6.2%–20.3% rate of congenital malformations, with neural tube defects most prominent. Teratogenic effects are dose-related with greatest risk at doses >1000 mg per day.	Relatively low excretion (0.68%); considered compatible with breastfeeding	Best to avoid in pregnancy unless absolutely required. High-dose (4 mg) folic acid supplementation recommended.
Antipsychotics			
Second-generation	Fewer data available, most showing no increased risk of malformations. Maternal hyperglycemia, impaired glucose tolerance, and weight gain may lead to maternal complications. Large-for-gestational-age infants reported. Floppy infant syndrome reported in clozapine exposure; monitor neutrophils in neonate for 6 months.	Excretion low, usually <3%, with exception of clozapine (Clozaril), which is seen in relatively high concentrations in breast milk	Overall, relatively safe in pregnancy; not treating serious mental illness in pregnancy poses greater risk. Most data with risperidone, olanzapine, quetiapine. Avoid clozapine in breastfeeding if possible.
First-generation	No increased risk of malformations seen with high-potency agents. Small increased risk with low-potency agents such as chlorpromazine (Thorazine). Transient extrapyramidal side effects; sedation; withdrawal symptoms in neonates.	Relatively low excretion reported although little data available. Sedation and parkinsonism effects possible in breastfed infants.	Haloperidol (Haldol), fluphenazine (Prolixin) favored during pregnancy because of long history of safe use and fewer hypotensive, anticholinergic, and antihistaminergic effects. Limited data in breastfeeding; relatively safe.
Antidepressants			
Bupropion (Wellbutrin)	No increased risk of malformation shown thus far	<1% excretion with no adverse outcomes reported	Well-characterized and considered reasonable option. May also help with smoking cessation during pregnancy.
Duloxetine (Cymbalta)	Little data	No published data, though exposure is low	Other agents with more data favored
Levomilnacipran (Fetzima)	No data	No published data	Other agents with more data favored
Mirtazapine (Remeron)	Sparse data, but one small study suggests no increased rate of major malformation	Low excretion; compatible with breastfeeding	May be useful also for pregnancy-associated emesis, insomnia
SSRIs	Controversial data regarding cardiovascular malformation with first-trimester paroxetine (Paxil) exposure. Larger and more recent studies show no overall increased risk for malformations with SSRIs. Conflicting reports with some showing decreased gestational age, low birth weight, poor neonatal adaptation, low Apgar scores (some of which could be due to underlying depression or anxiety). Conflicting reports regarding SSRI use in later pregnancy and persistent pulmonary hypertension (PPHN). Neonatal toxicity reported as transient jitteriness, tremulousness, and tachypnea. No problems detected in behavioral or cognitive development—greatest data with fluoxetine (Prozac).	Relatively low excretion, varies by agent: Fluoxetine: 3%–9% Paroxetine: <4% Sertraline (Zoloft): <2% Citalopram (Celexa): 5%–10% Fluvoxamine (Luvox): <2%	Best-studied and most-used class of psychotropics in pregnancy. Relatively safe in pregnancy; avoid paroxetine if possible. Sertraline results in lowest fetal drug exposure and lowest (undetectable) levels in breastfed infants; may be considered favored SSRI. Paroxetine use most controversial. Fluoxetine less favored for breastfeeding due to long half-life and active metabolite; disturbed sleep, colic, irritability, poor feeding reported.
Tricyclics	Relatively large database; recent meta-analysis of 300,000 live births revealed no increased risk of malformations. Neonatal anticholinergic effects. Transient neonatal withdrawal symptoms reported.	<1%–5% excretion; appear relatively safe during breastfeeding, with possible exception of doxepin	Well-characterized and considered reasonable options. Desipramine (Norpramin), nortriptyline (Pamelor) preferred due to lower anticholinergic and orthostatic hypotension risks. Monitor baby for sedation in breastfeeding.

Medication	Pregnancy	Breastfeeding	Recommendations
Venlafaxine/desvenlafaxine (Pristiq)	Earlier data regarding major malformations reassuring, but one more recent study suggested a possible association with birth defects; additional studies needed. Increased maternal blood pressure may be a concern during pregnancy, particularly at higher doses.	2%–9.2% excretion; no adverse outcomes reported	Other agents with more data favored
Vilazodone (Viibryd)	No data	No published data	Other agents with more data favored
Vortioxetine (Trintellix)	No data	No published data	Other agents with more data favored
Stimulants			
Amphetamines and methylphenidate	No apparent congenital malformations; may constrict blood flow to placenta, which reduces oxygen flow to developing fetus. May cause premature delivery, small-for-gestational-age and low-birth-weight babies; however, data inconclusive. Neonatal withdrawal possible.	0.2% excreted into breast milk; adverse effects usually not observed	Caution in pregnancy due to possibility of vasoconstriction and ability to disrupt blood flow to the fetus

Index

Trade names are capitalized, bolded page numbers are for fact sheets, and non-bolded page numbers are for quick-scan tables and general prescribing information.

A

Abilify, 49, **51,** 64
Abilify Discmelt, 49, **51**
Abilify Maintena, **51,** 63, 64
Abnormal Involuntary Movement Scale (AIMS), 123–125
acamprosate, 100, **102**
Adderall, 14, **27**
Adderall XR, 14, **27**
ADHD medications, 11–12
Adzenys XR-ODT, 14, **16**
Alpha adrenergics, 67
alprazolam, 69, 71, 132
Ambien, 71, 140
Ambien CR, 71
amitriptyline, 30, **44**
amphetamines, 14, 15, **16,** 131, 142
Anafranil, 30, **44,** 69
Antabuse, 100, **105**
Anticonvulsants, 67
Antidepressants, 29–31, 141. see also Tricyclic antidepressants (TCAs)
Antihistamines, 68, **72**
Antipsychotics, 47–50, 67, 141
    first-generation, 49, 63
    long-acting injectable (LAI) (see Long-acting injectable (LAI) antipsychotics)
    second-generation, 49–50, 63, 91
Anxiolytics, 67, 69–71, 140
Aptensio XR, 13, **25**
aripiprazole, 49, **51,** 63, 64, 131, 132
aripiprazole lauroxil, 63, 64
Aristada, **51,** 63, 64
armodafinil, 130, 132, 133, 134
asenapine, 49, **52,** 130, 131
Atarax, 70
Ativan, 70, 71, **75**
atomoxetine, 15, 17, 131
avanafil, 132

B

Barbiturates, 130, 132, 133
Belsomra, 140
Benadryl, 69, 140
Benzodiazepines, 67
    dose equivalencies, 71
    hypnotics, 68
    pregnancy and lactation, 140
Beta blockers, 67
Blood pressure parameters, 115–118
Body mass index charts, 119–122
brexpiprazole, 131
Brisdelle, 30, **40**
Bunavail, 100, **104**
Buprenex, 100, **103**
buprenorphine, 100, **103,** 132
buprenorphine/naloxone, 100, **104**
buprenorphine subdermal implant, 100, **103**
bupropion, 31, **32,** 130, 131, 141
bupropion SR, 31, **32,** 100
bupropion XL, 31
BuSpar, 69, **73,** 140
buspirone, 67, 69, **73,** 140
Butrans, 100, **103**

C

caffeine, 130
calcium channel blockers, 132
Campral, 100, **102**
Cannabinoids, 80
carbamazepine, 91, 92, **93,** 130, 132, 133, 140
Carbatrol, 92, **93**
cariprazine, 132
Catapres, **18,** 69
Celexa, 30, **33**
Central alpha agonists and antagonists, 68
Chantix, 101, **113**
chlordiazepoxide, 71
chlorpromazine, 49, **53,** 131
Cigarette smoke, 130
ciprofloxacin, 130
citalopram, 30, **33,** 130, 132
clarithromycin, 132, 133
clomipramine, 30, **44,** 69
clonazepam, 71, **74,** 132
clonidine, 15, **18,** 69
clopidogrel, 130
clorazepate, 71
clozapine, 49, **54,** 130, 131, 132
Clozaril, 49, **54**
codeine/hydrocodone, 131
Colloidal silver, 80
Complementary treatments, 79–81
    non-recommended, 80
Concerta, 13, **25**
Controlled substances, 134
Cotempla XR-ODT, 13, **25**
Cymbalta, 30, **35,** 141
CYP450 family drug interactions, 130–133

D

Dalmane, 71
Daytrana patch, 13, **26**
D-cycloserine, 80
Depakene, 92, **97**
Depakote, 92, **97,** 141
Depakote ER, 92, **97**
Depakote Sprinkles, 92, **97**
Deplin, 81, **82**
desipramine, 30, **44**
Desoxyn, 14, **23**
desvenlafaxine, 30, **34**
Desyrel (brand discontinued), 31, 70
Dexedrine, 15, **20**
Dexedrine Spansules, 15, **20**
dexmethylphenidate, 13, **19**
dexmethylphenidate XR, 13
dextroamphetamine, 14, **20,** 131
dextroamphetamine oral solution, 14
Diastat, 69
diazepam, 69, 71, 130, 132
diphenhydramine, 69, **72,** 131, 140
disulfiram, 100, **105**
Dolophine, 100
donepezil, 131, 132
Dopamine norepinephrine reuptake inhibitor, 31
Doral, 71
doxepin, 130, 131
doxylamine, 69, **72,** 131
Drug interactions, 127–133
duloxetine, 30, **35,** 130, 131, 141
Dyanavel XR, 15, **16**

E

Edluar, 71
Effexor (brand discontinued), 30
Effexor XR, 30, **45**
Elavil (brand discontinued), 30
EMSAM, 31, **41**
Epitol, 92, **93**
Equetro, 92, **93**
escitalopram, 30, **36,** 130, 132
Eskalith, 140
estazolam, 71
eszopiclone, 69, 132, 140
Evekeo, 14, **16**

Evzio, 100, **107**

F
FazaClo, 49, **54**
FDA label information, 137
Fetzima, 141
Fish oil, 79, 81, **86**
flibanserin, 132
fluconazole, 130, 132, 133
fluoxetine, **37,** 130, 131
fluoxetine DR, 30, **37**
fluphenazine, 131
fluphenazine decanoate, 63, 64
flurazepam, 71, 132
fluvoxamine, 30, **38,** 130, 131, 132, 133
Focalin, 13, **19**
Focalin XR, 13
Forfivo XL, 31, **32**

G
gabapentin, 69
galantamine, 131, 132
Geodon, 50, **62**
Ginkgo biloba, 79–80
Growth and body mass index charts, 119–122
guanfacine, 12, 15, 18, **21,** 67, 68, 70, 132
guanfacine ER, 15, 70

H
Habitrol, 101
Halcion, 70, 71
Haldol, 49, **55**
Haldol decanoate, 49, **55,** 63, 64
haloperidol, 49, **55,** 131
haloperidol decanoate, 63, 64
hydroxyzine, 70, **72**
Hypnotics, 68, 69–71, 140

I
iloperidone, 131, 132
imipramine, 31, **44,** 70
Inderal, 70, **77**
Informed consent guidelines, 126
Intermezzo, 71
Intravenous immunoglobulin (IVIG), 80
Intuniv, 15, **21,** 70
Invega, 50, **58**
Invega Sustenna, **58,** 63, 64
Invega Trinza, 50, **58,** 63
isoniazid, 130

J
Jornay PM, 13, **25**

K
Kapvay, 15, **18**
ketoconazole, 130, 132, 133
Khedezla, 30, **34**
Klonopin Wafers, 69
Klonopin, 69, 71, **74**

L
Lab monitoring, 135
Lamictal, 92, **94,** 140
Lamictal CD, 92, **94**
Lamictal ODT, 92, **94**
Lamictal XR, 92, **94**
lamotrigine, 91, 92, **94,** 140
Latuda, 50, **56**
levomilnacipran, 132, 141
Lexapro, 30, **36**
Librium, 71
lisdexamfetamine, 15, **22**
lithium, 91, 92, **95,** 140
Lithobid, 92. **95,** 140
L-methylfolate, 79, 81, **82**
Long-acting injectable (LAI) antipsychotics, 63–65
lorazepam, 70, 71, **75**
Low-dose naltrexone (LDN), 80
loxapine, 131, 132
Lunesta, 69, 140
lurasidone, 50, **56,** 132
Luvox (brand discontinued), 30, **38**
Luvox CR, 30

M
Magnesium, 80, 81, **83**
Melatonin, 68, 79, 81, **84,** 130
Metadate CD, 14, **25**
Metadate ER, 13
methadone, 100, **106,** 130, 131, 132
Methadose, 100, **106**
methamphetamine, 14, **23,** 131
Methyl B12 injections, 80
Methylin CT, 13
Methylin ER, 13
Methylin oral solution, 13
methylphenidate, **24,** 142
methylphenidate ER, **25**
methylphenidate transdermal, 13, **26**
metronidazole, 130
Minipress, 70, **76**
mirtazapine, 31, **39,** 67, 70, 130–132, 141
mirtazapine ODT, 31
mixed amphetamine salts, 14, 15, **27,** 131
modafinil, 15, 130, 132, 133

Monoamine oxidase inhibitor (MAOI), 31
Mood stabilizers, 91–92, 140
Mydayis, 15, **27**

N
N-acetylcysteine (NAC), 79, 81, **85**
naloxone, 100, **107**
naltrexone, 100, **108**
naltrexone, low-dose (LDN), 80
naltrexone ER, 100
Narcan Nasal Spray, 100, **107**
Neurontin, 69
Nicoderm CQ, 101, **112**
Nicorette Gum, 101, **109**
Nicorette Lozenge, 101, **109**
nicotine inhaled, 100, **110**
nicotine nasal spray, 101, **111**
nicotine polacrilex, 101
nicotine transdermal, 101, **112**
Nicotrol Inhaler, 100, **110**
Nicotrol NS, 101, **111**
Niravam, 69
Non-benzodiazepine hypnotics, 68
Noradrenergic and specific serotonergic antidepressant (NaSSA), 31
Norpramin, 30, **44**
nortriptyline, 31, **44**
NSAIDs, 130

O
olanzapine, 50, **57,** 63, 64, 130
Oleptro, 70
Omega-3 fatty acids, 79, 81, **86**
omeprazole, 130
Oral contraceptives, 132
Oral hypoglycemics, 130
oxazepam, 71
oxcarbazepine, 92, **96,** 130, 132, 133, 140
Oxtellar XR, 92, **96**
Oxytocin, 80

P
paliperidone, 50, **58**
paliperidone palmitate, 63, 64–65
Pamelor, 31, **44**
paroxetine, 30, **40,** 131
Paxil, 30, **40**
Paxil CR, 30
perphenazine, 49, **59,** 131
Pexeva, 30, **40**
Pharmacogenetic testing, 136–137
phenobarbital, 130
phenytoin, 130, 132, 133
pimavanserin, 132

prazosin, 70, **76**
Pregnancy and lactation, 138–142
Pristiq, 30, **34,** 45, 142
Probuphine, 100, **103**
ProCentra, 14, **20**
Prolixin decanoate, 63, 64
propranolol, 70, **77,** 131
ProSom, 71
Provigil, 15
Prozac, 30, **37**
Prozac weekly, 30, **37**
Pycnogenol, 80

Q
quazepam, 71
quetiapine, 50, **60,** 132
Quillichew ER, 14, **25**
Quillivant XR, 14, **25**

R
ramelteon, 68, 130
Remeron, 31, **39,** 70, 141
Restoril, 70, 71
ReVia, 100, **108**
rifampin, 130, 132
Risperdal, 50, **61**
Risperdal Consta, 50, **61,** 63, 65
Risperdal M-Tab, 50, **61**
risperidone, 50, **61,** 63, 65, 131
Ritalin, 13, **24**
Ritalin LA, 14, **25**
Ritalin SR, 13, **25**

S
S-adenosyl-L-methionine (SAMe), 80, 81, **87**
Saphris, 49, **52**
Sarafem, 30, **37**
Secretin, 80
Selective serotonin reuptake inhibitors (SSRIs), 30, 67, 141
selegiline, 130
selegiline transdermal, 31, **41**
Seroquel, 50, **60**
Seroquel XR, 50, **60**
Serotonin norepinephrine reuptake inhibitors (SNRIs), 30, 67
sertraline, 30, **42,** 130
Serax, 71
sildenafil, 133
Sonata, 70, 140
St. John's wort, 80, 81, **88,** 130, 132, 133
Strattera, 15, **17**
Sublocade, **103**
Suboxone, 100, **104**
suvorexant, 133, 140

T
tadalafil, 133
tasimelteon, 130, 133
Tegretol, 92, **93,** 140
Tegretol XR, 92, **93**
temazepam, 70, 71
Tenex, 15, **21,** 70
Tetrahydrocannabinol (THC), 80
thioridazine, 131
thiothixene, 130
Thorazine, 49, **53**
Tofranil (brand discontinued), 31, 70
topiramate, 132
Tranxene, 71
trazodone, 31, **43,** 70, 131, 133, 140
triazolam, 70, 71, 133
Tricyclic antidepressants (TCAs), 30–31, **44,** 67, 131, 133, 141. see also Antidepressants
Trilafon, 49, **59**
Trileptal, 92, **96,** 140
Trintellix, 142

U
Unisom, 69

V
Valium, 69, 71
valproate, 141
valproic acid, 91, 92, **97**
vardenafil, 133
varenicline, 101, **113**
venlafaxine, 30, **45,** 131
venlafaxine ER, 30, **45**
Versacloz, 49, **54**
Viibryd, 142
vilazodone, 133, 142
Vistaril, 70
Vitamin A, 80
Vitamin D, 80, 81, **89**
Vivitrol, 100, **108**
vortioxetine, 131, 142
Vyvanse, 15, **22**

W
Wellbutrin, 31, **32,** 141
Wellbutrin SR, 31, **32**
Wellbutrin XL, 31

X
Xanax, 69, 71
Xanax XR, 69

Z
zaleplon, 70, 133, 140
Zenzedi, 14, **20**
ziprasidone, 50, **62,** 133
Zoloft, 30, **42**
zolpidem, 71, 133, 140
zolpidem low dose, 71
Zolpimist, 71
Zubsolv, 100, **104**
Zyban, 100
Zyprexa, 50, **57**
Zyprexa Relprevv, 63, 64
Zyprexa Zydis, 50

CPSIA information can be obtained
at www.ICGtesting.com
Printed in the USA
LVHW020507021020
667590LV00009B/63